Say What You Really Mean!

Say What You Really Mean!

How Women Can Learn to Speak Up

Debra Johanyak

ROWMAN & LITTLEFIELD
Lanham • Boulder • New York • London

Published by Rowman & Littlefield
A wholly owned subsidiary of The Rowman & Littlefield Publishing Group, Inc.
4501 Forbes Boulevard, Suite 200, Lanham, Maryland 20706
www.rowman.com

16 Carlisle Street, London W1D 3BT, United Kingdom

British Library Cataloguing in Publication Information Available

Library of Congress Cataloging-in-Publication Data

Johanyak, Debra, 1953-
Say what you really mean! : how women can learn to speak up / Debra Johanyak.
pages cm
Includes bibliographical references and index.
ISBN 978-1-4422-3005-7 (cloth : alk. paper) -- ISBN 978-1-4422-3006-4 (electronic)
1. Interpersonal communication. 2. Communication in organizations. 3. Communication in management. 4. Women--Psychology. I. Title.
BF637.C45J645 2014
155.3'3336--dc23
2014030096

Printed in the United States of America

This book is dedicated to the memory of John Holodnak, my father, who imparted to me the importance of seeking knowledge, and to the memory of my mother, Leone Holodnak, who taught her four children to put words to good use. From my sister, Rebecca Oberg, I have learned the beauty of subtlety and restraint, whereas my brother, J. Scott Holodnak, models the perfect blend of a direct manner with a polite approach. The memory of my brother, John, inspires me to continually choose my words wisely.

Contents

Preface

Say What You Really Mean! has evolved over many years of personal experience in dealing with people who do not express themselves clearly. That includes me, on occasion. Those whose language utilizes fuzzy descriptions, limited details, missing explanation, a puzzling tone, an unclear message, or mysterious silence have raised questions that I have long sought to answer about the ways in which we communicate. Sometimes I was the one who failed to clarify a time, a reason, or a purpose. I have used the silent treatment to good and bad effect. I have been the target of silence with no clue as to why. My questions to others have drawn vague replies, deepening the mystery of meaning, without further efforts from me for clarification.

Many times I have listened to friends complain that they don't know what someone expects of them. Or they lament that a supervisor on the job has given unclear instructions.

"Why don't you ask for more information?" I suggest.

Their answers range from worrying about making a bad impression to having asked three times but are still receiving unclear information.

I hear loved ones make business phone calls who fail to ask the right questions. They come away with limited information and various uncertainties. "Call back," I urge them. "Explain the whole story. Get all the facts."

In the workplace I've witnessed miscommunication that leads to mistakes and occasional conflict. If we could just say what we really mean instead of adhering to restrictive social policy or failing to speak directly, we could enhance communication so that it becomes more productive.

This book is my attempt to call attention to ways in which women communicate indirectly. There are a variety of reasons why this happens, but becoming aware and taking steps to speak directly can enrich verbal interaction for improved results. As we learn to speak up in appropriate ways, we can more quickly and effectively explain goals and obtain desired results.

From teenagers to business professionals, women can learn how to change the way they express themselves and become more goal oriented. This book's ten chapters address ten issues that explain how and why indirect communication can go amiss. Each chapter includes Suggested Strategies for communicating more directly to get better results.

This book would not have been completed without the generous assistance of several professional editors and reviewers. I would like to acknowledge the instrumental editorial feedback from Charles Harmon. His patient guidance and keen eyes identified areas that needed clarification or enhancement. Robert Hayunga provided excellent production guidance and assistance in moving the manuscript toward publication.

I hope that readers will find useful ideas on how to identify and change indirect communication patterns to become more effective communicators. The knowledge I have acquired over many years I offer to readers in hopes of clarifying their personal and professional interactions.

Acknowledgments

Say What You Really Mean! is published with the help of several professional associates, good friends, and beloved family members whose input and assistance have contributed greatly.

Charles Harmon was instrumental in guiding the development and completion of the manuscript. His thoughtful attention to detail and timely reminders helped to keep the project on task.

Practical and technical support is indispensable. Robert Hayunga was readily available to answer my frequent questions and provide necessary information during the production process.

Michael Johanyak offered insightful direction to useful sources on the role of semiotics in social communication.

Sarah M. Carafelli designed the facial figures that are included in several chapters to illustrate important communicative principles. Her artistry, which adds a creative interpretive component to this work, is appreciated.

Discussions with my sister Becky, brother Scott, and children Jason, Matt, Stephen, and Bethany, have rendered much food for thought on this topic.

Introduction

Why Don't We Say What We Mean?

Most of us spend a fair portion of each day trying to express ourselves meaningfully to others. We share information, ask questions, make requests, and issue commands. But often it can seem like others just don't really understand what we're trying to say. They might get part of it, but they don't respond in the ways we want them to. This book is designed to help you come across clearly to others and achieve your personal and professional goals.

Generally, we hit the message mark more often than not. If someone fails to catch our meaning or fails to follow through as expected, we patiently resign ourselves to explaining things one more time or trying a different mode of expression. But let's face facts: It's frustrating when someone doesn't "get" it. After the second or third attempt, patience wears thin. You want to scream, "I can't say it any plainer than that!"

But many times we could and should speak more clearly. In fact, the way something is said can interfere with what is said and cause static in the communication flow. Each day we navigate conversational exchanges that can benefit from a direct approach based on a foundation of honesty. Even brief dialogue can be handled in ways that build up or tear down a relationship. Closeness can be cultivated in commonplace interactions where our lives intersect.

Let's use a popular example: A woman wants her husband to take out the trash after dinner. Yes, it sounds like a stereotype, but as we all know, most stereotypes contain at least a grain of truth. There he sits, ensconced in his living room easy chair watching football—oblivious to her washing dishes in the kitchen. Knowing he will raid the refrigerator at halftime, she bags the garbage and sets it beside the refrigerator to catch his attention.

Halftime comes and there he is, burrowing into the fridge as expected. But something goes wrong. He ignores the bag. Sandwich in hand, he heads back to the chair to watch the rest of the game.

She decides to hit him straight up and call from the living room doorway to be heard above the television:

"Honey, will you take out the trash?"

"Sure thing," he mumbles, taking another bite of the ham and cheese.

So she waits—and waits. The game ends. He watches the news and then heads off to bed.

"'Night," he calls from the stairs.

She starts to call him back with "Wait!" But suppressing the panic-stricken note from her voice, she mentally shrugs and surrenders the battle. What's the use? The same scene has played out dozens of times, and she always loses.

How can he leave that stinking bag sitting indoors all night? By morning the kitchen will reek. With a sigh, she grabs the trash and sets it in the garage. Then she joins her spouse in bed and pretends to be too tired to respond when he reaches for her.

"What's wrong?" he mumbles, his turn to be frustrated.

"Nothing," she sighs from her side of the bed, refusing to turn and face him.

Oh, there's plenty wrong. But no one's talking about it. So tomorrow when he grudgingly moves the trash from the garage to the outside receptacle, she will give him the cold shoulder at breakfast and perhaps maintain her chill into the evening as well, just to make him a little uncomfortable for his insensitivity. After all, she's not angry so much about the trash as about his ignoring her request for help.

Great communication? She punished his thoughtlessness so he'll remember the next time, right?

Maybe. Maybe not.

Generally, men are linear creatures. They prefer following a nice straight line from point A to point B rather than connecting the dots. Just ask them to do something—nicely—and most will do it, especially if it makes sense and doesn't infringe too far on their turf or time.

If we replay the preceding scenario, a more effective way to get her husband to take out the trash might resemble the following.

"Honey, can you take out this trash *now* so it doesn't *stink up* the kitchen?"

"Can I do it at half-time?"

This time she leaves a note on the fridge for half-time or pleasantly reminds him when he makes that sandwich. The bit about the odor should help because no one enjoys a smelly kitchen, especially when looking for a snack.

If he manages to forget despite her practical approach, she should let the garbage sit inside overnight to treat him to the fruit of his nonlabor in the morning. One whiff and he might be more likely to remember next time. If she can't bear the odor, she can take out the trash that night and the next day ask him to return the favor.

Adding nonverbal support to your words heightens their effect. The next time you ask your spouse to do something, approach and face him directly, making nonconfrontational eye contact—just enough to get his attention. Depending on both of your personality types, you can take his hand, smile, or rub his shoulder to make the request more palatable. Linking a positive action (physical touch) to a negative message (request a favor) can double your effectiveness and increase the chance of accomplishing your mission.

The goal is to be direct by asking hubby to take out the trash and explain why it needs to go tonight. Make sure he hears you clearly and understands what you are asking him to do. Try not to sound commanding or threatening. Most people don't like doing things just because others think they should. Offering a reasonable—and brief—explanation can help to ensure that the listener understands the nature of your request. Compliance often follows.

Using silence and body language as punishment usually is not effective. A person may get the point and do as directed. But no one will appreciate the accompanying tension each time miscommunication occurs and expectations remain unmet.

Situations like these may escalate over time, leaving spouses frustrated and affecting other areas of the relationship in negative ways. Intimacy can dwindle. Trust shrinks. Romance fizzles. Polite and caring coworkers and friends start looking like pretty good alternative companions . . . all because you don't press the point of making your request clear and direct.

You might be thinking, "What's so hard about taking out the trash?"

At times, all of us fail to grasp others' wishes as expressed in language or nonlanguage. Let's say your husband asks over breakfast for you to pick up a tube of antibiotic cream at the grocery store that evening while doing your weekly shopping. You get off work at five, head for the store, consult your mental shopping list, and proceed to the checkout without a thought for the antibiotic cream. Your husband meets you at the garage door and asks about it.

"I forgot," you mutter, only slightly apologetic.

He shows you a two-inch gash on his arm from the electric hedge trimmer that was covered by the pajama tops that morning. It's red and puffy.

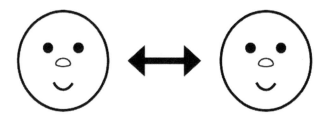

Figure 0.1. Balanced two-way communication

"Why didn't you tell me you were hurt?" you ask, exasperated. If you had known about the wound, you surely would have remembered to get the ointment.

Maybe he didn't want to worry you. Maybe the gash didn't look that bad to him. Now one of you will have to make another trip to the store for the ointment. Whoever it is won't be happy.

That extra little bit of communication can make life simpler!

Getting familiar with your mate's communication style often facilitates interactions between the two of you. If you realize he tends to give you just the basic facts of a situation, ask questions to get the rest of the story. If he forgets things, write a note or send a text reminder.

INNUENDOS

Communication is more than words. A comprehensive message embodies language, attitude, expression, and even physical actions. When the message is well crafted and transmitted efficiently, good things happen. Even bad news can be made palatable when packaged in a thoughtful manner.

Timing and location are key factors to promoting healthy communication. You don't want to "corner" your teen in the car on the way to soccer practice to reprimand him for a messy room. Nor should you invite your boyfriend of six months to a fine dining establishment to break up with him. Both situations can be handled more directly and with honesty-laced respect in a private area where you can express yourself openly without fear of being overheard.

Say What You Really Mean focuses on ways in which people can learn to communicate more directly with each other to accomplish their goals. Although it may seem logical to withhold or downplay difficult information, that tactic may not serve your interests or those of your listener. There certainly are times to be still . . . and others when you should speak up. In the chapters to come we will discuss these distinctions.

Here is a self-quiz to glean more insight about your style. Review the following list to see which statements apply and respond with a mental "true" or "false" reply:

- I sometimes hold back information that could hurt someone's feelings.
- I get frustrated when people don't tell me the whole truth.
- I don't know how to explain difficult situations.
- I feel like people don't really listen to me or care about what I say.
- I say as little as possible that might provoke others.
- I have to nag people to get things done.
- I often raise my voice or use a stern tone to get people's attention.
- I find myself repeating things to get others to listen to me.

- I wish I could speak more honestly and assertively.

If you responded "true" to several of these statements, this book can help you identify problem communication behaviors and teach you to build effective skills. Subverted communication can create obstacles to reaching your goals. Find out what you can do to remove those obstacles and create a clear path to success.

IS HONESTY ALWAYS THE BEST POLICY?

Although it's true that some things are best kept quiet, most relationships flourish with regular doses of honesty — not the brutal kind that wants its way no matter the outcome, but the kind that is thoughtful to others with a carefully planned goal in mind. This introduction looks at ways in which people can speak indirectly to each other without realizing it and become frustrated as a result. Becoming aware of indirect communication patterns is the first step toward change.

Chapter 1, Tell It Like It Is, explores the ways in which honesty can make a genuine difference at home and at work, build respect, and help to achieve personal and professional goals. First, find out if you are being honest with yourself and what to do if you are not. Then explore the ramifications of honesty and dishonesty in interpersonal relationships. Learn when it is best to "grin and bear it" in regard to a partner's bad habit, for example, and when to truthfully discuss negative aspects of your relationship or situation. Find out why sometimes it's better to deal with sticky subjects rather than hiding behind a veneer of complacence.

SHOUTS OF SILENCE

Spiteful words can hurt your feelings but silence breaks your heart.
—Anonymous

Chapter 2, Silence Loud and Clear, explores the pros and cons of "the silent treatment." Silence is a powerful tool that is often wielded as a weapon. Although keeping quiet in tense situations can provide a protective mantle of self-preservation, extending silence unnecessarily can bury important information under a shroud of misunderstanding.

Like extra-strength medication, keeping quiet may soothe agitated conversations that threaten to burst out of their restrictive boundaries. But like any medicine, too much can prove lethal, slowing the pulse of a two-way exchange to a flat-line finish. The right dose of silence given in an appropriate context can benefit relationships of every kind. But you have to measure and apply the dose carefully to make it effective.

Think about the times you have used silence to manipulate someone. Was it intentional? How long did it last? What response did it receive?

Chances are you haven't given much thought to when or how you chose to be silent. It just happened. Maybe you angrily withdrew or felt shut down. Whatever the reason, becoming aware of your "silent treatments" will allow you to use them constructively. Don't let short- or long-term verbal withdrawal happen by chance. Knowing when to stay quiet or speak up can have a powerful effect on your communication style.

TRUTH OR DARE

What you do speaks so loud that I cannot hear what you say.
—Ralph Waldo Emerson

Honesty is the topic of Chapter 3. It explains the importance of telling your listeners the truth without alienating them. This means being honest in a way that is good for others even if it is difficult for you. In trying to deliver a negative message or avoid the truth, your body can betray you with subtle signs and hints that listeners can pick up on, which can compromise your credibility.

Don't underestimate others' ability to accept truthfulness in unpleasant situations. Of course, someone under the influence of stress, medication, or other factors may not be able to competently handle the truth. But don't be afraid to say what you mean to the extent that your hearers will be able to understand you. Learn how to soften the blow of "bad" news (such as a poor sales report or a relationship problem) and get the audience on your side instead of creating tensions within the group by ignoring key facts.

FUNNY LITTLE FEELINGS

Sense and Sensitivity is the theme of Chapter 4. Should emotions lead or follow our words? Much depends on a given situation. Unlike controlled logic that maintains an orderly place of distinction in the human mind, feelings can run amok in the soul, creating havoc and general disorder in response to a charged situation. They burst forth into words and gestures that require restraint. Wisdom and self-control help a person to harness emotions in productive ways.

If your boss tells racial jokes that offend you, it is a good thing to let him know so he can be more aware of and responsible for his behavior. But how should you tell him? Generally, hurling curses or screaming insults will not help, even though that might be exactly what you feel like doing. Arrange a meeting where the two of you can sit down for a few minutes after lunch (one of the best meeting times) and privately discuss his comments.

Chapter 4 looks at ways in which we allow emotions to shape verbal and nonverbal language. When your boss calls you into the office for a reprimand, how should you respond? If a boyfriend wants to date others, what will you say? What impact does your emotionally guided response have on the ultimate outcome of a relationship? This chapter helps you become more aware of your emotional responses and suggests strategies for managing them.

HIS VIEW/HER VIEW

Are men and women really that different? At heart, aren't we all the same?

Chapter 5, His Fault/Her Fault: It Started in Eden, examines the role of direct communication in bridging the gender communication differences. Being indirect seems to be more of a female trait, which leaves men scratching their heads and trying to figure out the eternal feminine mystique. Many men use a direct style of communication, which can leave women feeling dominated and unvalued. Understanding core differences help men and women to appreciate each other and promote healthier verbal exchanges at home and on the job.

CONTROL FREAK

Do you ever feel like pulling out all the stops to control a conversation? Maybe you feel powerless when someone displays subtle wit or a manipulative edge. Or perhaps you desperately need to make a point to "win" the argument. However we do it, forcibly commanding our listeners' attentions through emotional ploys or witty machinations suggests we do not know how to let words speak for us to deliver a clear, certain message.

Chapter 6, Whining and Wheedling, describes common miscommunication situations in which we find ourselves using tactics such as whining, imperiousness, or teasing to lure a listener's attention rather than letting carefully chosen words do all the talking in a straightforward manner.

It is scary to feel out of control in a conversation, especially if it turns into an argument. But if you can harness emotions and use language constructively, you can learn to get your point across without appearing overly aggressive or controlling.

BAD MESSAGE VERSUS BAD PACKAGING

The path of life is long and fraught with perilous circumstances. Sometimes we find ourselves in a situation where we must deliver bad news. Falling profits and ailing health are two difficult topics that often must be broached with others. Knowing what to say, as well as how, become vital concerns.

Chapter 7, Breaking Bad News, discusses ways to announce bad news in a direct manner without being unduly offensive or hurtful. Communication strategies connected to firing a subordinate or ending a relationship are examples explored in this chapter.

Packaging a message is as important as the message itself. Imagine opening a birthday gift wrapped in newspaper or soiled gift wrap. Maybe the box holding a beautiful pearl necklace is mildewed or partially crushed. Wouldn't that type of deformed packaging make you question the value of the gift as well as the gift-giver's purpose?

The same principle applies to communication. The most important words in the world can fall on deaf ears when they are phrased inappropriately or out of context. Picture a travel agent casually describing scenic wonders at an exotic locale. As the agent describes this wondrous place while eating an apple, glancing out the window, and losing her train of thought from time to time, you might wonder if the site is really worth seeing after all. Maybe you should wait for her to get really excited when describing another location.

Alternatively, relaying bad news should be done with sensitivity and tact. Although you do not have to make things seem better than they really are, you should not exaggerate the seriousness of a problem. Just stick to the facts in a polite manner and say the words that must be said.

MAXIMIZE MINIMAL CONVERSATIONS

Sometimes language is better understood when accompanied by a sign or signal. Words may become these signals, or they may be paired with a hand gesture or facial expression. Chapter 8, Signs and Signals, explains how signage impacts communication in society and how we can learn to interpret it.

Communicating honestly is as important as communicating effectively. Withholding or misrepresenting information, whether deliberate or unintentional, can have a disastrous effect. Learning how to take control of your words, silences, and spaces can make you a more strategic speaker whom others will appreciate and respect. Integrity goes a long way toward enhancing or discrediting a speaker's image. The guidelines in this book will help you get your point across without compromising your meaning.

When you say what you mean with your audience's needs in mind, you can enjoy greater success in achieving your desired outcomes. Building messages one word at a time lets you reach critical objectives to enhance your relationships and well-being.

Chapter 9, Say Less and Mean More, examines ways to trim excessive wordiness from our speaking patterns to establish more economical conversations. Although some people are more verbose than others, this is usually a personality trait. Using words like currency helps us to use language more strategically.

Chapter 10, Words on the Web, explores electronic communication media that are predominant today. Is an e-mail more effective than a text message? Are face-to-face meetings obsolete? Communicating electronically is changing the way we interact with others. This chapter explains some of the differences between live and digital interactions.

In the Conclusion, Make It Count is the theme. Whenever we speak, it is usually for a purpose. This chapter advocates the need for women to use the techniques explained in this book as they stand up and speak out to embrace their rights, beginning at home and extending into the global community.

Because clear communication is vital to any healthy relationship, and effective communication is one of the top three skills sought by most employers, use this book to learn how to speak your mind directly and inoffensively to save time and get things done.

ONE

Tell It Like It Is

"How are you doing?" an anxious middle-aged aunt questioned her young niece who had just gone through a relationship breakup.

"I'm fine, getting into a new routine. Thanks for asking," the twenty-one-year-old responded after her boyfriend ended their two-year relationship.

"That's good," Aunt Sally said doubtfully. As much as she wanted to prod the young girl into sharing her pain and grief, she had to wait until Kelly was ready to open up. "Would you like to have lunch next week?"

There was a pause at Kelly's end of the phone line. "Maybe. I have some college work to catch up on. I'll let you know."

Kelly didn't contact her aunt for nearly three months. By that time she was mostly through the difficult stage of healing from the broken relationship. She had spent many lonely nights in her dorm, crying and wondering why Greg had ended things. But she was determined to recover on her own without troubling friends or relatives. If Kelly had opened up to Aunt Sally, she would've been surprised, and possibly comforted, to learn that her aunt had gone through a similar experience in college. Not only that, but Sally had gotten involved with a support group where she had learned coping strategies for managing grief and depression, and she discovered that it was normal to experience a sense of loss and plummeting self-esteem after a breakup. All of this and more she could have shared with her niece. Kelly, however, suffered in seclusion, felt guilty for mourning, and hid it from those around her.

Learning to speak up and be honest requires courage—and practice. If we can't open up to loved ones about personal matters, how can we learn to be direct about professional issues or life-changing concerns? Most of us need at least one or two confidantes with whom to share our innermost feelings. A confidante can offer comfort, advice, or even a warning if needed.

Ironically, although technology has streamlined and increased various forms of communication, in many ways we are communicating less effectively than before. This chapter explores an interpersonal approach to meaningful communication and the ways in which cultural and emotional constructs create obstacles that inhibit direct interaction.

Families that become fragmented by separation or divorce, overseas jobs, military service, and hectic schedules are just a few causes of increasingly limited or disconnected communication. Despite the best of intentions, people can lose touch without meaning to, regardless of Skype, Webcam, social media, and cell phones. Recent studies like the following by John Cacioppo and colleagues have documented the fact that a sizable portion of the population, and women especially, experience loneliness routinely despite being connected to a social network:

> Analyses separated by gender suggested that loneliness spreads more easily among women than among men and that this holds for both friends and neighbors. . . . [W]omen are more likely to be affected by the loneliness of both their friends . . . and neighbors . . . , and their loneliness is more likely to spread to other people in their social network.

Women also reported higher levels of loneliness than men.

Going through the motions of being interconnected with others may have little impact on a person's psychological or emotional well-being. A popular businesswoman or stay-at-home mom may rack up hundreds of social media connections—and yet still feel alone when a crisis hits. There are some issues, such as a spouse suspected of infidelity, a child's failing grades, or a devastating personal illness, that most of us don't want to discuss on Facebook or Twitter, or with any of the numerous casual acquaintances we make through daily contacts.

So who do you call when you need a shoulder to cry on? Chances are you may not have someone who is physically close by or technically well connected that you can confide in on short notice. As we shall see later, texting and tweeting do not always adapt well to personal messages, whereas e-mail and social media lack the firm security boundaries that most prefer. With growing concerns about national surveillance and lack of privacy, it is becoming increasingly difficult to find a person, and the means, with whom to connect in a deeply meaningful and personal way.

A *Newsweek* article by Johannah Cornblatt titled "Lonely Planet" indicates the growing prevalence of individual isolation and loneliness:

Between 1985 and 2004, the number of people who said there was no one with whom they discussed important matters tripled, to 25 percent, according to Duke University researchers. . . . Studies have shown that loneliness can cause stress levels to rise and can weaken the immune system. Lonely people also tend to have less healthy lifestyles, drinking more alcohol, eating more fattening food, and exercising less than those who are not lonely. . . . Loneliness can be relative: it has been defined as an aversive emotional response to a perceived discrepancy between a person's desired levels of social interaction and the contact they're actually receiving.

In a country of 300 million people, it seems odd to think that so many feel alone, disconnected, and out of touch. It's no wonder that communication, when it occurs at all, can seem scripted, unclear, or incomplete, leaving others unsure of our true thoughts and motives.

VULNERABILITY ISSUES

When disaster strikes, it is good and sometimes necessary to share a loss with someone who understands and cares. It is even better to discuss it with a person who has gone through a similar experience and can offer valuable insight. But trusting others with our most delicate emotions is often challenging. We are reluctant to appear weak or needy. Sometimes we worry that a confidante such as a spouse or close friend will exploit a confidence that has been shared.

Brene Brown, vulnerability expert, discusses reasons why people today are hesitant to share confidences with each other: "One of the reasons there is such an intimacy deficit today is because we don't know how to be vulnerable. It's about being honest with how we feel, about our fears, about what we need, and, asking for what we need. Vulnerability is a glue that holds intimate relationships together."

Why are we afraid to reveal fear and pain? Modern life discourages face-to-face intimacy. We take to the Internet to post statuses, tweet news, and instant-message loved ones in fleeting words, complex acronyms, and cartoonish icons. We will examine the technological impact on direct communication in another chapter.

Other factors play a role. Failure to confide may be as a result of fear of judgment or criticism. The unflinching "I told you so" is passed down from one generation to the next to those confessing personal difficulties or failures. Revealing a weakness can result in censure or condemnation. Concerns about appearing foolish or becoming ostracized prevent some tortured souls from sharing their deepest longings and weaknesses. Many females, especially young girls, prefer to suffer in silence rather than air problems that may invite criticism by authorities or bullying by peers.

When considering how to share sensitive issues with someone who might not approve, the speaker may preface her comments by saying, "Please don't judge me for what I'm going to tell you. Just listen so I can explain what's bothering me." If the listener is unwilling to comply or jumps in with a harsh response, the speaker can simply say, "I realize this is difficult for you to hear. Let's discuss it another time" or "Let's not discuss it." Adopting a listener-sensitive attitude helps to preserve the relationship even if the issue cannot be openly broached.

Unwanted advice is another reason some women hesitate to express themselves. Caring friends and relatives are often eager to suggest solutions to perceived problems. However, some people merely want to vent without inviting others' opinions. They seek out a sounding board for exploring options. Being direct about preferences can enlighten the listener. It may be helpful to begin with an explanation of the goal, "May I share a problem with you? I don't really need advice right now, just a listening ear."

Differing beliefs can keep people from being open with each other. Conflicting moral codes or opposing values systems can erect barriers between two people who are trying to have a meaningful conversation. When one ventures to share a concern, the other may take up arms to push the speaker toward change.

As the conversation opens, the first speaker could say: "I know we have different beliefs about this issue, but it would mean a lot if you would just listen to my perspective for now."

When you let others know the type of response you're looking for, they will often comply. As a result of mutual honesty and respect, the relationship can develop even deeper roots. The speaker will learn that she is free to express herself without fear of unpleasant repercussions, and the listener can show she is willing to be objective. After all, unconditional friendship is based on the premise of extending understanding and affection to those with whom we disagree. Sometimes it is possible to remain friends, even if speaker and listener are at odds on a particular issue.

FINDING FRIENDS AND CONFIDANTES

The ability to talk frankly with a friend may become the basis for establishing an open, direct communication style that can be adapted to romantic and professional relationships. Finding a trustworthy soul in whom to confide has become more challenging in today's world. In generations past, rural and small-town families with numerous members worked together closely at home, or in nearby fields or in town, and often included several generations: grandparents, unmarried aunts or uncles, out-of-work cousins, and multiple children. Growing up in close-knit communities offered a range of prospective confidantes with whom to share profound secrets, earnest desires, or persistent fears. Children in large families of bygone eras shared beds and bedrooms, promoting a strong bond. In contrast, children today usually have their own bedrooms stocked with technology and toys of all kinds that keep them riveted to a monitor or screen instead of engaging in face-to-face interactions with siblings and peers.

Rural life has declined as more families have become urbanized and dispersed throughout mainstream society. Tight schedules and frequent relocations present obstacles to building long-term relationships that are havens for exchanging personal information and building emotional support.

As more women have joined the workforce over the past fifty years, whether as married joint financial provider, single mother, or independent career builder, they have less time to cultivate friendships and enjoy satisfying communication. Meeting for coffee or going to the gym are great ways to socialize. But brief encounters such as these do not necessarily provide significant intimacy or time to fully engage a pair of friends in each other's lives. As more women juggle career and children, many are finding less time to address their personal needs. Friendships get put on the top shelf as a future goal rather than remaining available as an accessible option; cultivating confidantes is more of a luxury than a necessity.

At work, coworkers may not be suitable confidantes. Women must be careful when building relationships while on the job. Being too friendly may be interpreted as unprofessional, whereas being reserved seems to suggest introversion or noncongeniality, neither of which is laudable in the public arena. Although some experts support on-the-job friendships as making work more enjoyable and less stressful, others urge caution, such as *Forbes* writer Susannah Breslin, who is quoted in an article by Carolyn Gregore:

> Still, many of us draw lines separating our work and personal lives, seeing friendship as something that happens outside of the office. *Forbes* writer Susannah Breslin, for one, has argued that female friendship shouldn't have a central place in our work lives. According to Breslin, trying to make friends in the office is one of three common ways that women undermine themselves at work.

Confiding in a colleague that you see every day can lead to awkward repercussions if the friendship fizzles. Or, if the coworker proves untrustworthy, everyone around the water cooler may get access to your private revelations. Likewise, if job roles change—one of you is promoted to a supervisory position—the friendship dynamic will likely change as well.

Thus, finding someone with whom to communicate openly can be challenging. In fact, it has become a lucrative business for those who claim to offer "good listener" skills. Many life coaches now include the epithet "confidante" among their Website lists of services. For an hourly fee, you can arrange a session with a professional listener who will gladly hear whatever you want to say and provide the requisite solace, guidance, or counsel.

Sex trade workers increasingly report being paid to listen or make conversation rather than perform physical acts. Phone and Internet "counseling" services offer "paid" conversation to lonely or busy people. Online Websites direct anxious visitors to listening services, or provide informal support for free, as reflected in this March 11, 2011, post on Ask.com: "How can I find someone to just listen to my problem and maybe advise me what to do?"

Licensed relationship counselors indicate a rising number of clients that now schedule appointments to discuss personal issues and get informal feedback when they have no one else with whom to share these concerns. An eighty-four-year-old divorced woman, Jackie, began seeing a therapist for depression. She made good progress through a few sessions and claimed to feel "wonderful" after each biweekly meeting, only reluctantly ending the visits when the therapist claimed Jackie was ready to be released from treatment. Jackie missed the sessions where she could talk nonstop for an hour to someone who actually seemed to listen. Similarly, a fifty-year-old divorced man, Todd, began seeing a counselor for anxiety after his wife left him. In the months that followed, he opened up to talk about other areas of his life, including a troubled childhood and a substance abuse addiction twenty years before. Even though the man had struggled with a mild speech impediment when younger that left a residual effect on his pronunciation, talking with the counselor increased his self-confidence and helped to minimize the impediment so that it became almost indiscernible. Over the course of therapy Todd joined a singles group and began doing volunteer work. He indicated that talking with the psychologist, an intelligent and compassionate woman in her sixties, made him feel more "valued" and "understood," and Todd continued to see the counselor until he passed away unexpectedly from a medical problem a few years later.

The ability to talk frankly with someone who is trustworthy can build confidence and courage that prepares one for more extensive and less personal communication. Consequently, the successful pattern of direct communication will likely come full circle and become self-perpetuating. Once you begin to speak up, you may never want to clam up again!

Clearly, people in general and women in particular have an innate need to connect in meaningful ways, and that need is not being fully met in contemporary society. One outcome of this problem is that women have less experience and support in speaking directly to others in public places. It's not unusual for the supermarket grocery clerk, bank teller, or soccer mom to unexpectedly open up to a complete stranger about her medical condition or marriage problem. I've experienced it countless times, and although it usually evokes empathy, sympathy, or even joy (for positive stories), I'm often puzzled by the readiness of women I've never met to share the most intimate parts of their lives with me — someone they don't know and may never see again. I do my best to be understanding and offer advice, condolences, or congratulations.

FEAR OF SELF-DISCLOSURE

Another obstacle to straightforward discourse is discomfort with self-disclosure. Professional counseling or therapy can be effective for certain individuals, but other women are hesitant to explore their innermost feelings with strangers, as indicated in this Web page discussion on fear of self-disclosure:

> People's decision to seek psychological help strongly correlates with their comfort about revealing personal thoughts or feelings to another person, according to a study published in the *Journal of Counseling Psychology* (Vol. 50, No. 3) by Iowa State University assistant psychology professor David Vogel, PhD, and University of Wisconsin-Milwaukee assistant educational psychology professor Stephen Wester, PhD. (Palmer)

Some women are hesitant to self-disclose to friends, having been raised to never discuss issues like money or sex with those outside the family. Consequently, they go through life keeping burdens a secret while maintaining a façade that all is well. Certain women have been raised with the idea that disclosing personal family secrets is dishonorable, a form of treachery that reveals a weak nature, and that strong character is modeled by a steely exterior that hides secrets within and keeps others out.

However, women in general are frequently team oriented. They find strength in numbers, so they prefer to share strong emotions and serious problems with close friends or relatives who may be able to help or at least provide stress relief and moral support. Generally, the ability to share personal information depends on the level of trust shared with a prospective confidante, as suggested by Michael Draper and colleagues:

> Findings indicate that the more difficult it is to self-disclose, the greater impact it has on the friendship (Collins & Miller, 1994; Morry, 2005). Therefore, disclosing in-depth about difficult topics should have the most influence on the friendship. Previous research (Buhrke & Fuqua, 1987; Collins & Miller, 1994; Fehr, 2004; Morry, 2005) has found that, regardless of the level, self-disclosure is positively related to friendship closeness and satisfaction. This has important implications for friendships. Disclosing to a friend can lead to a greater liking of the friend (Collins & Miller, 1994). Disclosure also communicates the desire of the discloser to attain a more intimate, or closer, relationship (Collins &

Miller, 1994). (3–4) . . . There is a certain amount of trust required for people to share vulnerable issues with others, and this trust generally exists only between close friends.

Concern about potential gossip and betrayal are other reasons why some women hold back from confiding in others. Even trusted friends and beloved family members can let a secret slip, intentionally or otherwise, sometimes with catastrophic results. Social networking among teens provides strong evidence that the risk of mockery, ostracism, and threats may prevent young girls from confiding in classmates or neighborhood friends. Even if it doesn't happen to them directly, witnessing the horrific effect on peers can be an effective deterrent against revealing personal information in a public forum. This learned reservation is likely to follow young women dealing with self-esteem issues and thus inhibit them from self-disclosing.

Although keeping a journal or diary is helpful in encouraging people to explore innermost thoughts and feelings, these written accounts are not meant to be shared. It is in learning to interact in verbal ways with others that we learn to speak up in professional settings.

FEAR OF REJECTION

Fear of rejection plays a huge role in the decision of whether to confide in someone, and if so, whom. Confessing mistakes, broken relationships, embarrassing medical conditions, or financial setbacks can be traumatic for those who worry they will be viewed as failures. This concern is legitimate because some people avoid those with known issues like these. Confiding in someone about a delicate situation requires tact and finesse, as well as sound judgment in selecting a trustworthy confidante.

When a girl on the playground invites a few classmates to join her on the swings and they refuse, she will be less likely to invite them another day, fearing more rejection. Similarly, when a female employee on the job offers a great idea, which is rejected by others, the employee may feel rejected. But if she is emotionally mature and reasonably confident, she will probably continue to make suggestions in the future. Learning how to handle rejection ideally should occur at a young age. Unfortunately, for some women who have experienced more of life's downs than ups, that may not be the case. As a result, they tend to withdraw or speak more indirectly.

In the professional realm, some women are insecure about being themselves. They feel that they are expected to live up to someone's beliefs about who they should be, not who they really are. This perception fuels indirect communication that reveals only partial or obscure facts, an idea supported by a recent *Forbes* article by Glenn Llopis on workplace fear:

Too many people fear that they can't be themselves at work. Unfortunately, this is a growing sentiment amongst employees as the workplace becomes more diverse each year. Everyone wants their authentic identity to be accepted. Employees are tired of feeling stuck between who they really are and what others want them to be. As a result, they believe they can't deliver their full workplace potential. . . .

To overcome this fear, you must view your uniqueness as a source of strength—not a weakness. People will embrace your unique identity the moment they know that it has value. If you don't value yourself, how can you expect others to value you? Take the time to educate others about what naturally makes you unique and how it influences the ways you think, act and innovate—as well as the results you can generate.

Because women have been active in leadership roles only for a generation or two, many are still finding a place and forging identities that capitalize on their education and experience. Any hesitancy in defending her right to a unique viewpoint can cost a female her authority. She must be willing to stand up for what she believes in—especially herself. Being honest about who we are and what we want is paramount. From that point on, women can learn to speak up about anything that impacts their personal relationships or professional situations.

PRACTICAL PRESSURES

In addition to personal and emotional impediments, some women avoid speaking up at work as a result of worry over losing their jobs. Because the owner, manager, supervisor, or boss is the authority figure, most women understand the importance of following rules and showing respect. Just as important is a woman's fear of losing her job for being too direct. As women continue to enter the workplace and climb the corporate ladder, they can take comfort in knowing that as indicated by information from the Fact Sheet on Professional Women: Vital Statistics, more positions are being filled by women than before.

- The number of women in the labor force is projected to be more than 78 million by 2018.
- About 73 percent of working women had whitecollar occupations in 2009.
- Today most mothers—even those with the youngest children—participate in the labor force.

Women who work to build an independent career, contribute to a multi-income household, or function economically as a single parent may be less likely to speak up to authority figures at work, fearing loss of job or denial of promotion as retaliation. Financial worries and family needs often influence women to avoid making waves by speaking up in ways that could annoy management or challenge coworkers. They are more likely to keep their opinions to themselves than to take a chance on saying something that will make them stand out in a negative way and potentially jeopardize their job status or future progress.

SOCIAL ATTITUDES AND CULTURAL CONDITIONING

The women's movement of the late twentieth century encouraged women to stand up and speak out on their own behalf or on behalf of others in need. Although more women today are less hesitant about expressing their views, those that hold traditional views or that are socially or culturally conditioned to be compliant or reserved may have difficulty in being forthright.

Given the increasing frequency and means of communication, it would seem likely that people would be less shy and more outgoing than in the past. But some research indicates the opposite, as explained by Karen Payne on her Web page of the Caltech Counseling Center:

> The number of people reporting some form of shyness has been gradually increasing over the years. The most recent research suggests that at any given point in time, close to 50% of the general population report that they currently experience some degree of shyness in their lives. In addition, close to 80% of people report having felt shy at some point in their lives. . . . The most typical situations that often trigger this kind of reaction are ones involving authority figures (teachers, administrators, leaders, etc.), potential one-on-one romantic or intimate encounters, having to initiate action in a group setting, or initiating social action in unstructured settings. These kind [sic] of situations often elicit reactions at one or all of the following levels: cognitive, meaning thoughts; affective, meaning feelings, physiological, meaning within the body; or behavioral, resulting in a withdrawal from the difficult situation. . . . In addition, cultural changes within the United States, such as increased crime forcing children off the streets and smaller families resulting in fewer siblings and smaller peer groups, are thought to be influences resulting in children growing up with less opportunity for unstructured interpersonal development.

Payne suggests forms of treatment that go hand-in-hand with learning to communicate openly:

> The first and most important step in overcoming shyness is finding the right person to talk to. A skilled mental health professional can be very helpful in assessing the degree to which your shyness is effecting [sic] your well-being and can help you determine whether or not shyness is really the problem, versus some other type of emotional difficulty (anxiety, depression, etc.). Once properly assessed, the counselor or professional might suggest several options: individual counseling, group counseling, or medication. . . . Behavioral interventions include recog-

nizing the kinds of behaviors that result in avoidance and working on engaging in more active initiating kinds of behaviors that will result in increased contact with others.

Many women are programmed by their upbringing or religious training to avoid conflict through submissive attitudes toward parents, spouses, and authority. Others come from backgrounds where it is considered impolite to disagree with others or offer differing viewpoints. When confronted, they will make conciliatory gestures or walk away, refusing to engage in disharmony. These women maintain the status quo and prefer blending in with the crowd rather than standing out as a target.

Some women have been taught that it is wiser—and safer—to comply. For example, a forty-five-year-old caregiver of a father with dementia reluctantly had him admitted to a nursing facility when she and her family could no longer provide around-the-clock care for his growing needs. Connie visited every day at first and then gradually tapered her visits to a weekly schedule. When she discovered one Sunday that her father was still unwashed and in his pajamas at 1 p.m. because of a staff shortage, Connie became distressed and hesitantly asked an aide about helping her father to wash up and get dressed. The aide explained that help was short, so Connie assisted her father before leaving at three p.m. when the second shift of nursing staff arrived.

Connie went home, tired and depressed, questioning whether she had done the right thing by placing her father in a nursing home.

"Did you tell them he needed help?" her husband asked over dinner.

"Yes, but I didn't push it, because I was afraid they would take it out on him after I left."

Mothers of young children often voice similar concerns. Although they will raise questions or even complain about the lack of quality care provided by a daycare employee or a teacher, some mothers will not do more unless the problem becomes serious, fearing reprisals against their children. That is not a response typically voiced by fathers, however, who are often more aggressive in dealing with daycare and school concerns. We will examine in greater depth the differing communication styles of men and women in another chapter.

Flirting is another social behavior wherein women may be more indirect than men. Although in general females are much more forward about expressing interest in a man than they used to be, some are accused by the men with whom they flirt of wearing "masks" and not being "transparent" about their feelings. Consequently, their meta-communication, or body language, may be far more revealing than their words.

At a club, for example, a young lady might wear revealing clothes, eye-catching makeup, and a strong scent to catch the attention of a man that interests her, and she will likely be successful. Furthermore, she may consciously or subconsciously use body gestures like touch, eye contact, smiling, and physical proximity to reveal her attraction. But if the pair actually has a conversation, her words may adopt an aloof tone or she may play verbal games about her interest, unwilling to be perceived as "easy" or "loose."

Although such behavior is universally recognized as flirtation, it leaves many men perplexed as to the woman's true intent. Is she merely seeking masculine attention? Does she want to be admired? Is she insecure about her beauty or femininity and need to be reassured? Or is she fishing for a hookup?

A thirty-five-year-old man working at a nonprofit organization was approached by an attractive thirty-three-year-old coworker who frequently praised his job skills and friendly personality. She would wrap her arms around his neck and make flirty statements while standing behind his chair in the cubicle. When he asked if he could call her, she gave him her phone number. Soon after, the man sat down with her at the company cafeteria during a lunch break and noticed that she seemed friendly but less forward. When he called her a day later, they talked for several minutes before she ended the call. The man was surprised and dismayed when the following day the department supervisor took him aside and asked him to stop "harassing" the female colleague.

> "But she showed interest in me," he explained, "and gave me her number. Other employees saw her flirtatious behavior—you can ask them."

Rather than get further involved with the situation, the supervisor told the male employee it would be best to avoid the coworker. The man was shocked that his colleague had initiated interest, given him her number, and then involved their supervisor. For the next few days the female stayed away, but within a week she came and again stood by his desk, apologizing and placing a hand on his arm. The man was polite but suggested that they not talk any more because apparently there had been a misunderstanding. The woman frowned but respected his wishes and kept a discreet distance with only an occasional remorseful glance his way as she passed the cubicle.

Although this woman's behavior may seem to suggest she has emotional or perhaps even psychological issues, it is not uncommon for some women to flirt and withdraw by turns, as though being coy. A couple of generations ago, girls were raised to be reserved if not aloof with boys until a suitable one properly asked her on an acceptable date—approved and possibly supervised by her parents.

Today, the traditional dating practices that evolved over the early twentieth century have diverged in numerous directions that are far removed from the original model. However, some confusion about appropriate male and female behavior remains. A girl who flirtatiously attracts a man's attention may feel that once she has achieved that objective, she can now move on to the next target. Other ladies have second thoughts once they attract a man's romantic interest and back off to discourage further attention. Another possible reason for a woman to evade a man with whom she has been flirting is that in the current social climate of confused sexual mores and potentially risky outcomes of sexually transmitted diseases (STDs) and unwanted pregnancies, she might have second thoughts about how the mutual attraction should proceed.

Whatever the reason, most women are unwilling to tell a guy directly, "I don't want to go any further with this; sorry for wasting your time." Rather, with a smile and a wave she heads back to the dance floor to look for another chance encounter where she can again exercise her alluring powers or remain secure in the protection of her "posse"—the girlfriends she is with—so that she cannot be singled out for individual attention by a man she no longer finds attractive.

On a broader scale, the rules of flirting and dating continue to transform at a rapid pace. Women of all ages are confused by expectations: theirs, the man's, and society's. When does flirting become teasing and potential become a promise? When their bodies become the "playing field" of the dating game, women are too often the losers and end up sacrificing their self-esteem, their personal freedom, their health, and their authenticity. From the moment of attraction, women must find ways of comfortably, yet directly, expressing their preferences and relational goals. Otherwise, they will continue to serve as silent slaves—just as women have for millennia—to the expectations of male partners and uncertain directions.

As we have seen, many women fail to clearly articulate what is important to them in every area of life, from being honest with themselves and family members to voicing specific feelings and goals in relational contexts, and withholding concerns and convictions in public venues like the workplace. Here in the twenty-first century women have earned the right to have their say at last. They cannot let anyone—including themselves—get in the way of being clear and direct about what they think.

In the chapters that follow, we will consider a range of subversive communication behaviors that hinder conversations at home or in public. In learning how to overcome barriers to effective communication, women can begin to use language as the powerful tool it is to build bridges that lead to more harmonious relationships and successful outcomes.

SUGGESTED STRATEGIES

1. Consider finding a confidante or mentor with whom you can share important information. Of course, you will determine the level of self-disclosure that is comfortable for you. As you open up with others, you will likely become more forthright about your thoughts and feelings.
2. Look for ways to express your opinions on public matters. Write a letter to the editor or communicate with your government representatives about issues of concern.
3. Reflect on the ways in which you communicate directly and indirectly with others. Are there times when speaking up more directly could be beneficial?
4. If your communication style feels restrictive, consider how you can change to become more outspoken in suitable ways. In other words, you don't need to adopt an in-your-face attitude, but you may want to be clearer about your views.
5. Do you know women who refrain from speaking openly? If so, should they be encouraged to be more direct? How might you encourage them to do so?

REFERENCES

Bouris, Karen. "How Vulnerability Holds the Key to Emotional Intimacy." *Spirituality and Health* 1 Nov. 2012. Web.

Cacioppo, John T., James H. Fowler, and Nicholas A. Christakis. "Alone in the Crowd: The Structure and Spread of Loneliness in a Large Social Network." *Journal of Personality and Social Psychology* 1 Jan. 2009: 977–991. 984. Web.

Cornblatt, Johannah. "Lonely Planet." *Newsweek* 20 Aug. 2009. Web.

Draper, Michael, Rachel Pittard, and Michael Sterling. "Self-Disclosure and Closeness." Hanover College, 18 Apr. 2008. Web. 7 Oct. 2013. http://vault.hanover.edu/~altermattw/social/assets/w08papers/Draper_Pittard_Sterling.pdf.

Gregore, Carolyn. "Why You Should Care about Having Friends at Work." *Huffington Post* 9 July 2013. Print.

"How Can I Find Someone to Just Listen to My Problem and Maybe Advise Me What to Do?" *Ask.com*, 11 Mar. 2011. Web. 23 Oct. 2013. http://www.ask.com/answers/6435081/how-can-i-find-someone-to-just-listen-to-my-problem-and-maybe-advise-me-what-to-do.

Llopis, Glenn. "Getting Past 4 Common Workplace Fears." *Forbes* 24 June 2013. Web.

Palmer, A. "Self-disclosure a leading factor in not seeking therapy." American Psychological Association, 1 Sept. 2003. Web. 7 Oct. 2013. http://www.apa.org/monitor/sep03/factor.aspx.

Payne, Karen. "Caltech Counseling Center." Caltech Counseling Center, n.d. Web. 25 Oct. 2013. http://counseling.caltech.edu/general/InfoandResources/Shyness.

"Professional Women: Vital Statistics." Fact Sheet 2010: Department for Professional Employees, n.d. Web. 24 Oct. 2013. http://www.pay-equity.org/PDFs/ProfWomen.pdf.

TWO

Silence

Loud and Clear

As indicated in the previous chapter, language can be used either as a powerful tool or as a deadly weapon. Learning to use words in either manner requires patience, time, and effort. In conjunction with verbiage, however, we must consider the implications of silence—intentional silence—and its coordination with spoken language to enhance or diminish the communication process.

Most of us choose to be silent at times for a variety of reasons such as annoyance, fatigue, or uncertainty. However, strategic silence is used to manipulate the meaning between the words found on either side of a verbal void. Unspoken communication sometimes leads to serious consequences and should be used with caution.

WOMEN AND HISTORICAL SILENCE

History reveals some interesting things about women's communication—or lack thereof. Ancient records suggest that women's words were neither shared publicly nor recorded for posterity at nearly the rate that men's were. The patriarchal tradition grew out of the fact that men experienced public life much more openly than women, and consequently, men, rather than women, recorded community events through the historical lens of male perspective. This *enforced silence* ensued because women were not culturally encouraged to speak publicly throughout much of recorded history, nor were their words considered significant.

When acknowledged at all in public records, women were typically mentioned for criminal acts or domestic duties such as marriage, housekeeping, and child-bearing. Women who did speak up with distinctive views were deemed lawless, immoral, and even insane, an impression that lingers today:

> Women who speak out, women who go against the grain, women who question the system, women who have emotions, women who express themselves, can be very easily tagged with a psychiatric diagnosis that can be extremely difficult to get rid of. Many of the diagnoses applied to women involve conditions considered "dangerous." A woman might be a "danger to herself and others," so she can be committed, yes, involuntarily. Family members, guardians, law enforcement, all of these people can make the decision to commit a woman on the basis of her psychiatric history, even if a diagnostic label was not applied properly.
>
> Many people are surprised to learn about the tangled and complex history of psychiatrisation and the ways in which it has been used to silence, marginalise, and oppress women. Unfortunately, many of these same people are unaware that the same tactics used in 1600 are still being used today, albeit under different names. . . . (Smith)

Yet, silence is not always a negative restriction placed on women. In recent generations, silence has served as a refuge and a haven for those unable to speak for themselves, as explained by Jane L. Parpart, "[s]ilence and secrecy also have a long history as survival strategies for women (and men) in marginal positions." She goes on to say:

> While silence and secrecy can be symptomatic of passivity and disempowerment, as well as a means for reinforcing gender hierarchies, as we have seen, they can also provide the space for discovering and consolidating inner resources, questioning the status quo, and developing long-term strategies for renegotiating gender relations. At an individual level, silence and secrecy can protect women from disempowering contexts where their voices have no institutional or collective power. Silent vigils and the use of appropriate symbols can reinforce group identity, build collective strength, and subtly challenge oppressive behavior (9).

Thus, although silence is not necessarily a bad thing, the potentially negative implications should be kept in mind. Likewise, the prospective positive applications cannot be dismissed.

In premodern literature, women were frequently silenced. Female characters that were enabled to speak or made their views known were the "dark ladies" of ill repute, whereas the "fair ladies" tended to be understated and insipid. Heroines in the writing of William Shakespeare and Edgar Allan Poe, if we accept these authors as representative of their respective eras, depicted "good" women as mainly passive and reserved and "bad" women as outspoken and aggressive. Shakespeare's strongest heroines are very direct, and they die tragically; Cleopatra defies Rome and denounces lover Mark Antony by killing herself rather than being conquered; Juliet rebels against her parents' choice of husband by pretending to die and then committing suicide; mad Ophelia sings lamenting songs about women's sexual victimization before drowning. In Poe's short stories, none of the principal tragic heroines (Ligeia, Morella, Berenice, Madeline) speak directly but are rather shadowy figures that seem surreal and yet ultimately triumph over the men who try to control them. Whether Poe was depicting these women as victims or victors (a debate still conducted by critics today), he nevertheless represents them as tragic for their inability to communicate directly.

Nineteenth-century author Nathaniel Hawthorne represents his most famous heroine, an adulteress named Hester Prynne in *The Scarlet Letter*, as a strong and admirable woman who is given her "say" in the seventeenth-century Puritan community where she resides. However, as a result of her moral emancipation, she is branded by her sin forever. For women, there was a price to be paid for being outspoken in word or deed. As a result, silence emerged as a protective cocoon to keep women—real and literary—hidden from public life and social criticism.

WOMEN'S CONTEMPORARY SILENCE

Finding a voice and using it constructively has become an overarching goal for twenty-first-century women. Therefore, silence should be used to good purpose and carefully evaluated for intent and outcome.

Silence, especially among women, takes many forms. One type is *elective silence*, or the conscious choice to say nothing. A second type is *extended silence*, or choosing not to speak for a protracted period of time. *Imposed* silence occurs when someone is forbidden from speaking or whose words are overridden by a legal code, patriarchal social norms, or a competing force.

Elective silence occurs when women choose to be silent as a form of psychological self-control or emotional separation. Refusing to interact with a family member during conflict is a way of establishing boundaries or activating a protective shield against emotional pain. Some women lack the right words to express thoughts and feelings clearly during arguments, so they keep quiet. Others adopt an air of emotional distance by cutting off communication for a period of time. Sometimes people do this to incite curiosity or concern. Others do so to provide themselves with time to reflect, problem solve, or heal.

Extended silence is less common and more mysterious. People may consider a person who speaks little, or hardly at all, over a long period of time as abnormal. Why would a woman choose to indefinitely stop interacting with others? Is she hiding her innermost thoughts or afraid her words will be dismissed? Perhaps she feels disconnected from those around her, considering herself on higher or lower moral or social ground.

Most commonly, silence is practiced as a way of protecting what one really thinks. This can be done to spare someone's feelings or because the nonspeaker doesn't know how to respond. But failing to speak up can lead to misperceptions or an emotional implosion—with disastrous results.

My friend Lisa shared this story of how silence caused problems early in her marriage. Here is my retelling of the incident (with her permission).

> "I hope you like the roses I got you for our anniversary," her husband Jeff offered confidently, handing the bouquet to her as he entered the back door after work.
>
> "They're nice," she told him, gritting her teeth. "They look very—cultivated."

Inside, Lisa was seething. For her, hothouse flowers held all the appeal of gumball machine jewelry. She loved garden mums and hand-picked daffodils. But florists' roses left her cold—and irritated.

After a year of marriage, Lisa felt her husband should know this. Hiding her disappointment, she said nothing and pretended to enjoy the roses. But she took the first opportunity of revealing her displeasure during their next argument, which "coincidentally" erupted that evening.

> "Don't you know I hate hothouse flowers?" she snapped in a transition from the conflict at hand to feelings she had hidden at first. "They're artificial! Anything else would have been better."
>
> Jeff's face reddened. "I can't read your mind! Tell me what you want. No—better yet—make a list."
>
> "That's so romantic," Lisa bristled sarcastically. "You should KNOW what I like by now."
>
> "How—by osmosis?" Jeff stomped off to the family room to watch TV.

The couple's celebratory evening ended with the roses ejected into a trashcan and a cold wall of silence erected between them.

Thus began the couple's first lesson about indirect communication. If before the anniversary Lisa had explained to Jeff the type of gifts she enjoys, or if Jeff had asked her preferences, their argument could have been avoided. Several months later, with the help of a few counseling sessions, Lisa promised Jeff to be clearer about her likes and dislikes, and she apologized for being insensitive to his well-meant efforts. Jeff said he would learn more about Lisa's preferences and ask if he wasn't sure.

Failure to speak up can lead to misunderstandings. It's always better to discuss an issue than skirt it and risk miscommunication.

Ironically, silence often speaks louder than words. We feel uncomfortable around someone who doesn't speak, and we try hard to understand what *isn't* being said. In our communication-sated culture, those who keep to themselves do not easily fit in because most of us use language to accomplish many things: getting to know someone, doing our jobs, obtaining knowledge, and so on. Words are the relevant currency of personal and professional interaction, making a living, and other daily activities.

ACTIVE SILENCE

Sometimes loading the air with unspoken tension is a choice of weapon in a battle for relational control. Deliberately not speaking, or "active silence," is the most obvious way to withhold information and disable interaction. Sometimes people keep quiet to avoid tension, or at other times, to create tension. Being quiet can have a similar effect as screaming, depending on the person at whom it is directed. We often view silence as a passive behavior, but it can convey a strong attitude.

If you are talking to someone with little to say, you'll probably wonder what that person is thinking. Is she listening intently or withdrawing emotionally? As friends become comfortable with each other, they settle into an easy silence at times when neither is expected to speak; they just enjoy the moment. But it takes time to reach that level of mutual comfort with nonspeaking.

The other end of the silence spectrum involves couples who are quite familiar with each other and use silence as punishment. One gets annoyed and clams up. When asked "What's wrong?" the nonspeaker shrugs or says "nothing," leaving the other person confused and apprehensive. The silence may be complete, including the refusal to answer questions or make small talk, such as "Pass the salt." In other cases, the silence extends only to purposeful dialogue, and the nonspeaker may interact casually with the other person. The "rules" vary. The nonspeaker will resume speaking only after getting her way or when she decides silence is no longer necessary. Her partner may get the point and do as expected to reduce tension and restore normalcy.

Research suggests that ignoring someone or responding with silence affects the same nerve centers in the brain as those impacted by physical pain. Thus, giving someone "the silent treatment" causes similar stressful reactions in the body as physical punishment. A *Purdue University News* article indicates that the "cold shoulder"—sometimes called "ostracism"—is widely practiced, with negative results:

> When a person is ostracized for even a brief period of time, the anterior cingulate cortex, the part of the brain that detects pain, is activated. . . . The people who are ostracizing often feel a strong sense of belonging with each other, as well as feeling empowered. . . . People who are excluded react one of two ways. The most common reaction is to try to improve a person's characteristics or behavior so they are included or fit in. Or, people who are excluded frequently become destructive and vindictive. (Neubert)

The "silent treatment" can be found across cultures and socioeconomic strata. According to Lisa Zadro, who interviewed several victims of ostracism, this type of silence can leave a lasting detrimental effect on the "targets" (recipients):

> These interviews opened my eyes to the fact that forms of ostracism, such as the silent treatment, were being used to devastating effect in homes, businesses, and schools around the world. The stories that these people shared with me were often extraordinary. Some were unexpected; for instance, one woman claimed that her husband had trained the dog to ostracize her and had wanted advice on how to get the dog's attention back. (I recommended visiting a vet for training advice and, in the meantime, filling her pockets with bacon.) Other stories were simply heartbreaking. One young woman in high school was ignored by every single one of her classmates for several months. She found this widespread, unremitting ostracism so distressing that it led her to attempt suicide. Many targets reported experiencing ostracism episodes that lasted years, even decades, from their loved ones, primarily parents or spouses. These targets lamented that receiving the silent treatment from their loved ones meant that they dreaded going home at night—their homes were a place of ongoing distress and angst rather than a refuge from the outside world.

Many mental health professionals and family or relationship counselors believe that "the silent treatment" is a serious form of emotional abuse, as indicated by counselor/therapist Patricia Jones:

> Just about the worst form of abuse is the Silent Treatment . . . someone who is in the same room as you are, but who is acting like you don't exist. They don't speak to you, they do not answer your questions or make comments on your statements[;] they completely ignore you and act as if you are invisible. And it works because nothing makes us madder than someone who we KNOW hears us, sees us, and knows without a shadow of a doubt that we exist, act as if we are not even there! We feel a "rage" rising from somewhere deep inside of us when we are ignored. . . . I believe the silent treatment is the worst form of emotional abuse. It is, in all reality, a punishment because it makes you feel like a non-person, who is not valued or cared about. . . . It is really

all about CONTROL. . . . Silent treatment is a form of torture to someone that they profess to love . . . it allows the abuser to avoid any confrontations, any uncomfortable questions or subjects that they don't want to talk about, and it gives them a way to get out of any accountability to their spouse.

Many women use language for pleasure as well as purpose. Several studies suggest they have a desire or need to express more words per day than men do. When a talkative person suddenly stops, it becomes quite noticeable. Family members against whom silence is directed become uncomfortable as a communication gap develops. By its nature, silence is mysterious. Until we become fully acquainted with someone—learning to understand conversational pauses, quiet moods, and sensitive topics— it is difficult to understand the person's use of silence.

Women sometimes keep silent for reasons that men do not necessarily share:

1. Low self-esteem. Some women feel out of place in traditional male-dominated environments. One example is a newly hired female employee, especially in a male-dominated occupation, such as construction or mining. Some women hired into these occupations have indicated reluctance to join in the male banter, which may be sexist, racist, or sexual in nature, until they gradually establish camaraderie on more neutral topics.

2. Control. A woman might choose to stay quiet when others, such as a child or spouse, depend on her for information. Using parental privilege or feminine mystique to attract attention that has been otherwise scant is a way to reassert her position and reawaken others' attention.

3. Disagreement or disapproval. Silence can signify withdrawal if the nonspeaker disagrees but is unwilling to voice dissent. For example, a young woman left her husband to stay with her mother while deciding how to handle marital problems. When the husband convinced her to return, the girl's mother said nothing directly, but her disapproval was evident from her brief suggestion that her daughter wait to return home until the weather improved, although the weather played no serious role in the issue. Eventually the daughter admitted she had sensed her mother's unspoken disapproval but had followed her own inclinations because her mother did not question her openly.

Understanding why women remain silent can equip those around them to better interpret and deal with the various causes. Often, giving a nonspeaker thirty minutes or so to be alone provides "down time" in which she can process her emotions and get back on track with everyday communication.

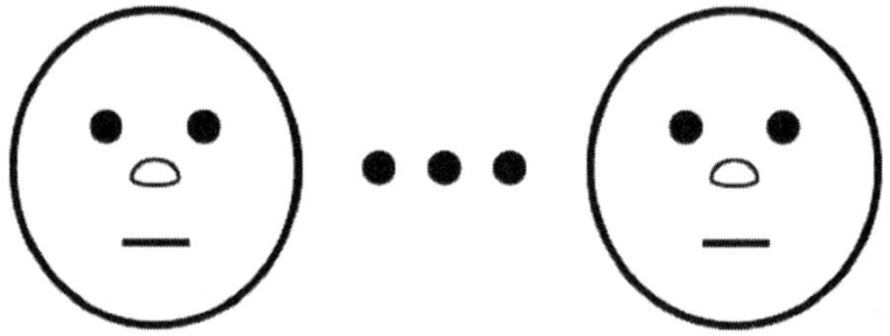

Figure 2.1. Silence and the communication void

When women become the targets of nonspeak, they seem to be especially perceptive in deciphering the unspoken code. One expert calls it "women's intuition."

> Research on nonverbal communication skill has clearly shown that women are, as a group, better at reading facial expressions of emotions than are men. As a result, women are more likely to pick up on the subtle emotional messages being sent by others. Women are also better at expressing emotions through their facial expressions, tone of voice, and body, particularly positive emotions. Men are better at controlling felt emotions and at hiding emotions behind a "poker face." There is also evidence that women are seen as more empathic than men, and that they are more likely to see themselves as empathic. In other words, women tend to be more "open" to others' emotional messages. . . . Where does this ability to read emotions come from? It has been suggested that it is mainly due to social power. Women, who have been historically lower in social power, spend more time observing and scrutinizing those in power (i.e., men, and powerful women), and become more attuned to their nonverbal cues. (Riggio)

Using built-in skills and generations of experience can help women to correctly interpret the silence of others. Learning to consciously hone this ability will likely enhance communication.

INCIDENTAL SILENCE

Not all silence is negative. In Western culture, verbal silence feels awkward. We talk freely every day through a variety of media, so silence within families seems unnatural. The silent sage image represents someone who budgets language as prudently as finances. At times it is best to listen before speaking; that's why we have two ears and one mouth. As our mothers used to advise, "If you can't say something nice, don't say anything at all." There is wisdom in verbal restraint. Still, choosing not to speak for any length of time will raise concerns in those around us.

Several years ago an American family lived in the Middle East where they raised a daughter for the first three years of her life. The girl learned to speak that country's language as her native tongue.

When the family returned to the United States, the child abruptly stopped speaking. She would cling to her mother and point to things she wanted. Her anxious parents sought a professional opinion, thinking something was wrong with a three-year-old who wouldn't talk. The expert explained the child was confused by the abrupt transition from one daily language to another. Although she understood her parents' spoken English, she had relied on Farsi for communication. The doctor told the parents to give their daughter time to adjust. Within two weeks the child began speaking English words, and within a month she was conversant in her "second language."

Like these parents, most of us are uncomfortable when someone stops speaking. Silence isn't considered "normal." Emotionally and culturally, we are trained from birth how to speak and what to say. When someone doesn't speak regularly, we assume something is wrong.

Yet, many professionals believe that selective silence is an intuitive communication tool with great potential:

> Silence doesn't get the attention it deserves. It is a powerful form of communication which we often use without thought. With a better understanding of its significance we can become better 1) communicators and 2) readers of a person's emotional state including, their intentions and how engaged they are. (Dawson)

In an article titled "Shyness Is Nice," authors Barbara Markway and Greg Markway question the negativity associated with not speaking:

> So what's so bad about being quiet? Why is it so difficult to accept, even embrace it as a source of strength? I believe a big reason is that it doesn't match the cultural ideal. For example, how many times have you seen a television show or a movie where the main character was reserved, cautious and thoughtful, and where this was seen as positive? Most often, the media portrays popular characters as outgoing. Quiet characters, when they are seen, often assume the role of a victim.

Speech patterns, mental or physical impairments, or health disorders may influence a speaker's use of silence. Interacting with these individuals requires added effort and risk of miscommunication. Most of us understand these conditions and interact effectively despite them. Similarly, some people are forced to work as diligently to communicate with those who can speak, but choose not to. Without spoken language, mutual understanding is harder to achieve.

PASSIVE SILENCE

Silence sometimes hides information. This is a form of silence in which a person speaks, but the language is empty of meaning. Vague words and abstract concepts provide little practical value. Double-speak in a political context is a popular example. We can all think of public figures who dance around sensitive issues by discussing unrelated problems.

Some people reveal partial information for many reasons. Using selective silence becomes detrimental when information is needed or deception is uncovered. Certainly, partial silence can obscure key issues, as well as call into question the speaker's motive.

A young man recalls coming home from school as a boy and entering the kitchen where his mother faced the sink, peeling potatoes. Without speaking, her stiff shoulders and apathy to his arrival sounded a silent alarm about her mood. He would rush to his room or play outdoors to escape the tension. Consequently, the boy grew up without fully understanding his mother's silence, which was not targeted at him, and we only learned later in life that she suffered from depression. If he had known when younger, he might have understood her better, and his self-esteem would not have suffered. Instead, he spent years wondering what he had done to upset her.

In another situation, a young teacher whose job performance exceeded school expectations, Jessica, received an e-mail from the department chair (Mrs. Parker) requesting her presence at a meeting that the assistant principal would also attend. Jessica e-mailed back to ask about the purpose of the meeting. Mrs. Parker e-mailed the cryptic message: "Departmental matters." Jessica was unsure whether to be elated or concerned. Why was the assistant principal going to be there? Would she be offered a special assignment? Or was she about to be fired?

The meeting was disastrous. The assistant principal politely indicated he was there only as an observer, although he interjected occasionally to support Mrs. Parker's claims that Jessica had ended summer classes early the year before. Jessica was dumbfounded. She took her teaching duties seriously. Because she had not anticipated these charges, she had come unprepared to defend herself. She began taking notes.

"Well?" Mrs. Parker asked impatiently as Jessica wrote. "Why did you release last year's summer school students early?"

"I didn't release them early," Jessica answered, surprised. "I'll check my records to find out what happened." That had been a whole year ago. She couldn't remember anything of consequence taking place then.

Mrs. Parker brushed aside Jessica's lack of ready knowledge as incompetence. Jessica simply must never do it again. So Jessica politely left the meeting, seething inside, hurt and misunderstood. The assistant principal had indicated this issue would not appear on Jessica's personnel record, but Jessica felt humiliated. When she reviewed her year-old files, she found that the previous summer the campus air-conditioning had broken down during a heat wave, and several instructors—Jessica included—had taken students outdoors to the patio area for the last hour of class, close to noon, when high temperatures made the building extremely uncomfortable. She was furious that Mrs. Parker had not explained her concern beforehand so Jessica could check her file before the meeting, when the assistant principal would witness her lack of defense.

Fortunately, Jessica continued to receive positive evaluations from her peers and was eventually promoted and tenured. But what could have been a productive mentoring relationship between new and experienced educators never materialized, and Jessica felt as though she was constantly under scrutiny until Mrs. Parker retired.

If only Mrs. Parker had told Jessica how to prepare for the meeting . . .

If only Jessica had pressed for more specific information . . .

Passive silence—the failure to disclose full facts—can be hurtful and harmful. Some women's careers depend on the quality and quantity of communication that is shared between colleagues.

Another type of passive silence is hiding true feelings and opinions, instead expressing views that seem compatible with those of others. On the surface we appear agreeable, but underneath we resent stifling ourselves.

Example: Two coworkers leave a presentation on hiring minorities.

"Didn't Jack act like a jerk at the meeting?" one employee says.

"I know what you mean," the other replies.

That's a noncommittal response. Is the second speaker saying she understands the first speaker's point—or agrees with it? Such comments keep the speaker in a neutral position, but they prevent an open exchange of viewpoints.

Here's a more productive version:

"Didn't Jack act like a jerk at the meeting?"

"Do you mean his comment about the company not hiring minorities? I'm not sure what he meant. Let's ask him."

Another example of passive silence can be found in the acquiescent responder:

"Where do you want to eat lunch, Helen?"

"Wherever you want to go."

"What about that new sushi place?"

"Okay."

Fearing ridicule, Helen doesn't mention she dislikes sushi. When they order, she will have a side salad. Helen could have gotten better results by being direct:

"Where do you want to eat lunch, Helen?"

"I don't know what I'm in the mood for. How about you?"

"What about that new sushi place?"

"You know, I've never been fond of sushi. Is Napoli's okay instead?"

By ending with a question, she shows the first speaker that she is willing to negotiate. Her coworker does not have to guess what food that Helen likes or dislikes, and Helen does not have to suffer in silence at a restaurant she does not enjoy.

People in long-term relationships usually figure out the silences between the words. But sometimes they are not quite sure what a partner is trying to tell them. With the help of body language, they engage in a passive silence game, like this one between husband and wife:

"Bob, will you keep an eye on the kids while I go shopping?"

Behind his newspaper, Bob mumbles something that sounds like "All right."

"You sure?" his wife Joann asks.

An unintelligible response follows, so Joann pursues it. "Do you have something to do? Would you rather I wait until after dinner?"

The newspaper rattles, followed by a weak "Go ahead."

Uncertain, she lingers. "I can go another time, honey."

"That's okay." (Does he mean her offer to wait is "okay," or that she doesn't need to wait?)

Joann wrestles with interpreting Bob's attitude—low voice, lack of eye contact, mumbled words, vague meanings. If she goes and he doesn't want her to, will she later be met with a cold wall of silence? Or should she accept Bob's words at face value?

An honest response builds trust and promotes understanding while reducing tension. When we shroud words with vague meaning, others get confused. Using firm, clear language can save time and spare feelings.

Back in the 1930s, a teenager who lived on a farm begged her mother to let her visit "city" relatives in a neighboring state. Anna was permitted to go despite her mother's mild reservations; she took a bus to a small town in Pennsylvania and was met by her middle-aged uncle who hardly said two words on the drive home. In the small, neatly kept house with her uncle and aunt who were in their late forties, Anna noticed they never spoke to each other. The wife served meals punctually, setting well-laden plates on the table without a word. The husband ate silently, newspaper propped before him. Anna's misery grew as she realized they weren't talking to each other and said little to her. When the day came for her departure, Anna left as eagerly as she had arrived.

In this situation, not only did the aunt and uncle display active silence toward each other, but Anna's mother also used passive silence in failing to warn her about the couple's tension, which she knew of.

Active or passive silence is often symptomatic of a relationship problem. People who turn off their speech like a faucet to impact another person, especially in negative ways, have retreated so far into their psyche that language no longer seems valid for them. Silence becomes its own "second" language that takes time to learn and interpret.

Instead of wrapping our feelings in a protective blanket of silence, it is healthier to channel emotional distress into positive interaction. Recent medical and psychological research has shown that counseling and journaling can be therapeutic for patients suffering from chronic illnesses like cancer or arthritis. A randomized trial by Joshua M. Smyth and colleagues found that patients with mild to moderate asthma or rheumatoid arthritis "who wrote about stressful life experiences had clinically relevant changes in health status" at four months, compared with those in the control group. In another study, Maloni and Kutil studied the effect of "antepartum support group for women hospitalized on bed rest" and concluded that "an opportunity to talk in a confidential and supportive environment may be an important antepartum nursing intervention in helping them [women] cope." Sharing difficult emotions with others allows a hurting person to explore complex subjects in a safe and comforting way. Conversely, holding negative emotions inside has been shown to lower immune system function and increase stress levels.

Timing is essential. Sometimes it is good to restrain thoughts: "A prudent man keeps his knowledge to himself, but the heart of fools blurts out folly" (Proverbs 12:23). Most of us have done our share of blurting and hurting. But refusing to speak for an indefinite period of time suggests strong feelings are boiling under the surface—or perhaps hints at an emotional vacuum.

Let's suppose a newly married couple is having an argument. After several minutes they give up and head off to different rooms. Moments later the husband returns to his wife with the words,

"But you know I love you!"

How does the wife interpret this? If the conflict is about money, she might feel her husband is using passive silence (avoiding the topic of money) to deflect her from the argument. Or she may think he's "apologizing" through his declaration of love or trying to "conquer" her with emotion. He, on the other hand, may take her unremitting silence as intended "punishment" for him, while she actually may be reflecting on the conflict and sorting her feelings.

A timeout can be a great way to defuse tensions. But at some point it's important to return to the issue and find resolution, or agree to disagree amicably. Silence—even well-intended silence—can be a hindrance if productive dialogue is not resumed. Keep in mind that "passive silence" means we are not completely straightforward. We may exchange words but leave something unsaid, creating an implicit untruth.

SILENCE AT WORK

A generation or two ago, women were still relatively new to most public professions. Some women were able to become doctors, attorneys, and politicians before 1950—but in small numbers compared to men. As more female students enrolled in college and embarked on professional careers, they learned to navigate what was still in many ways "a man's world."

In the early 1980s, a renowned Midwest law firm with more than twenty attorneys hired its first female lawyer, eager to update its practice with women practitioners and acknowledge the 1970s' feminist advances. The female attorney remained at the law firm for three years, eventually relocating to a larger firm in Colorado. Interviewing the former firm's colleagues after her departure for how they remembered this courageous feminist trailblazer, the answer was nearly universal: her chronic use of profanity. Obviously this habit has nothing to do with silence—except to imply that this brilliant woman's success in the legal industry was overshadowed by her desperate need to fit in with male colleagues—all of whom routinely used profanity. Off-color language was her way of rising through the ranks to be accepted, instead of relying on her courtroom expertise, which was mainly swept under the rug in favor of more colorful accounts of her communicative prowess.

Recently I attended a meeting of about seven men and women where a disagreement evolved over a policy handed down by an administrator. An employee vote was needed on a new hire, and the (absent) administrator required that the vote be conducted in writing within a "live" meeting of a quorum of employees. The committee felt that an e-mail vote should be adequate, given everyone's disparate schedules.

A female employee suggested not telling the administrator how the vote was taken and simply send him the results. This represents an interesting example of "passive silence," where incomplete information would be shared.

A male coworker suggested going to the administrator's superior (i.e., "pulling rank"), which illustrates the male characteristic of using hierarchy to get things done.

Another female felt the administrator should be approached directly and "reasoned with." She used words like "we" and "our," revealing her sense of connectivity with other committee members. Although this represents a more direct approach, it also illustrates a largely female strategy of lateral problem-solving using "team" unity. No one's suggestion seemed to be more correct or insightful than anyone else's. In the end, the decision for how to proceed was postponed until the next meeting.

Recent studies about women's workplace silence as reported by psychologist Jennifer Hartstein in an MSN video report suggest that "many men can be vociferous . . ." and women lack courage while in large groups of men. Instead, female employees often "keep the peace" and "wait it out" rather than participating in a meaningful work-related discussion. Business executive Ivanka Trump agreed with Dr. Hartstein and added that women tend to be more collectivity oriented, often keeping quiet in groups with high numbers of men. Instead, women study body language for clues to gauge others' emotions and attitudes.

Another study reported similar findings. "Women who are outnumbered by men in a group are less likely to speak their mind. In fact, new research has found that women speak 75 percent less than men when in such a setting" (Mielach). Many women found strength in numbers rather than independently:

> When voting by majority decision, women deferred speaking if outnumbered by men in a group. However, when voting unanimously, the researchers found that women were much more vocal, suggesting that consensus building was empowering for outnumbered women. . . . "Women are less likely to be viewed and to view themselves as influential in the group and to feel that their voice is heard." (Mielach)

For this study, *The American Political Science Review*, an academic political science journal, published the findings in which researchers studied 94 groups with five or more people each.

RELEASE FROM SILENCE

In other parts of the world, many women still have no public voice. When they do speak up, their words are given little consideration in patriarchal societies. One example relates to child marriage. According to a World Vision study released in March 2013,

> more child brides are being led into arranged marriages due to an increase in global poverty and crises. Parents who live in fear of natural disasters, political instability and financial ruin look to arranged marriages as a way to save their struggling families. Every day, 39,000 girls younger than 18 will marry. . . . "Women have no rights to give an opinion in the family," Humaiya, a 16-year-old from Bangladesh who managed to escape marriage, told *The Huffington Post* in March [2013]. "My father didn't listen."

Humaiya's story is not uncommon. Many women around the world feel that their identity as a person and their worth as a female is ignored or challenged by family patriarchs or local authorities. These women are struggling to overcome imposed silence by gathering publicly, marching in demonstrations, displaying banners, and blogging on the Internet. Their voices are finally being heard to alert surrounding nations in a call to action.

Recent news reports have proliferated of women struggling under imposed silence as victims of assault while in military service, as farm workers, as undocumented immigrants, or simply as wives and mothers in domestic abuse homes. Some of these victims practice elective silence in refusing to confront their abusers for fear of repercussions or because they lack the knowledge or means of recourse. Women victims of inequity, assault, and discrimination must band together to find strength in numbers while seeking redress.

Silence demonstrates self-control and emotional repression, which can be good or bad. Those who want to communicate in meaningful ways should use silence proactively or sparingly.

SUGGESTED STRATEGIES

1. Practice what you want to say while alone, before a meeting, so you can go prepared to speak up with confidence.
2. Ask the person who is organizing the meeting to add you to the agenda so your information will be expected.

3. Work on building confidence by refusing to be defined by restrictive labels like "shy," "unassertive," or "reserved."
4. Use active or passive silence sparingly and for good purposes.
5. Interpret others' silence carefully to avoid misunderstandings. If in doubt, ask questions.

REFERENCES

Dawson, James R. "Communicating through Silence." ADI Marketing, 9 Aug. 2012. Web. 20 July 2013. http://amarketing.com/2012/08/09/communicating-through-silence/.

Goldberg, Eleanor. "Yemeni Girl Who Evaded Child Marriage, Says She'd 'Rather Die' Than Get Married Off." *Huffington Post* 22 July 2013: Video.

Jones, Patricia. "The Silent Treatment: A Form of Abuse." Dove Christian Counseling, n.d. Web. 31 July 2013. http://www.dovechristiancounseling.com/SilentTreatment.html.

Maloni, J. A. and R. M. Kutil. "Antepartum Support Group for Women Hospitalized on Bed Rest." *AM J Matern Child Nurs* 25: 204–10. *NCBI*. Web. 9 July 2013.

Markway, Barbara and Greg Markway. "Shyness is Nice." *Psychology Today* 28 Aug. 2011: n. pag. Web.

Mielach, David. "Silent Women: Why Women Don't Speak Up." *Business News Daily* 20 Sept. 2012: n. pag. Print.

Neubert, Amy Patterson. "Cold Shoulder, Silent Treatment, Do More Harm than Good." *Purdue University News*, 27 July 2005. Web. 15 July 2013. https://news.uns.purdue.edu/html3month/2005/050727.Williams.exclusion.html.

Parpart, Jane. "Choosing Silence: Rethinking Voice, Agency, and Women's Empowerment." Gender, Development, and Globalization Program. Center for Gender in Global Context, 1 July 2010. Web. 20 July 2013. http://gencen.isp.msu.edu/documents/Working_Papers/WP297.pdf.

Riggio, Ronald E. "Women's Intuition: Myth or Reality?" *Psychology Today* 14 July 2011: n. pag. Web.

Smith, S. E. "Psychiatrisation: A Great Way To Silence Troublesome Women." this ain't livin', 13 Aug. 2010. Web. 22 Apr. 2013. http://meloukhia.net/2010/08/psychiatrisation_a_great_way_to_silence_troublesome_women/.

Smyth, Joshua M., Arthur A. Stone, Adam Hurewitz, and Alan Kaell. "Effects of Writing about Stressful Experiences on Symptom Reduction in Patients with Asthma or Rheumatoid Arthritis: A Randomized Trial." *JAMA* 281: 1304–1309. *JAMA Network*. Web. 2 July 2013.

Why Women Don't Speak Up At Work. Perf. Jennifer Hartstein, Ivanka Trump. MSN youtube, 2013. Film.

Zadro, Lisa. "Silent Treatment: Uncovering the Nature and Consequences of Ostracism." *Association for Psychological Science Observer* 26: 768–74. *Association for Psychological Science Observer*. Web. 1 July 2013.

THREE

Is Honesty Always Best?

"I didn't hit the trashcan," twenty-four-year-old Emily giggled to her middle-aged friend and neighbor Jane as they stood on the sidewalk, staring at the car.

"Yes, you did! I just watched you," Jane laughed, giving her friend a playful shove.

After leaving her driveway and hitting the trashcan, Emily had pulled her Honda CRV to the curb and was checking the back bumper for damage. A six-inch scratch was the only telltale sign of the mishap.

"Brandon will never notice. Don't tell him," Emily implored her neighbor.

"I won't tell him, but you should. He'll be mad if he finds out you were dishonest about it," Jane said.

"But he won't find out," Emily insisted. "I'll get it fixed before he sees it."

Jane shook her head. She wouldn't keep secrets like that from her husband. Why couldn't Emily just tell Brandon what happened?

Indeed. Why do many women hide the truth about negative events from husbands or boyfriends? Interestingly, some women worry that the men in their lives will be critical or mocking. These women try to guard themselves against their mate's irritation. They don't want to make a bad impression or reinforce a negative perception, as indicated in this *Parenting* article:

You see, we have different ideas on bedtime. I also conceal my dollar-store toy purchases (he hates "landfill junk" in our home) and the amount I spend on their birthday parties.

I don't think of myself as a liar; I think of myself as a normal wife, sidestepping and spinning to keep the peace. And I'm not alone: "I keep things from my husband all the time," says Angela, a mom of two in Connecticut. "I just don't want him thinking I'm too much of a softie, say, if the kids broke something or didn't do their chores."

But I've learned that leaving your partner out of the loop consistently means there's a problem. "If there's an agreement you're constantly breaking, you either need to stop or get rid of the agreement," says Stephanie Coontz, director of research and public education for the Council on Contemporary Families (CCF). Try to get down to an irreducible set of rules that you both agree have to be done consistently, and allow for slight variations in other areas.

Why are we so tempted to whitewash the facts? It's often because our values don't jibe. (Ralston)

Although many of us keep from spilling the whole truth at least occasionally, we can agree it's not a good idea to hide things very often. What if Brandon were to ask Emily outright about the car? If she lied, would deception sink even deeper into their relationship? Would she become angry by his challenging question? If he doesn't ask, is it "ethical" for her to avoid telling him?

Most people will agree that there are lies of commission and lies of omission.

The first type, *lies of commission,* refers to stating something that isn't true. This is an overt action of verbally speaking, suggesting, or supporting an untruth. Telling your mother-in-law that little Sarah got all As on her report card when in fact your daughter actually earned Cs would be an act of commission—outright deception.

The second type of untruth involves *lies of omission,* that is, keeping silent about something that is false. When your mother-in-law asks how her granddaughter is doing in school, and you reply, "She's earning good grades," meaning she's doing as well as she can by earning Cs; this could become a deceptive act of omission if you know the grandmother will interpret the statement as your daughter is earning As. It all boils down to intent.

Being honest with ourselves and others is an important way of speaking directly.

SELF-DISHONESTY

Aggressive dishonesty involves going to great lengths to create nonfiction. Examples include someone who creates a false persona on a social networking Website, or a woman who dresses or acts in a certain way to create a specific impression that may not be her true self. An extreme variation of this type of deception is the woman who fools herself into believing she is pregnant when she is not and then steals another woman's baby to raise as her own. Similarly, a woman who seduces a married man may convince herself that she is leading him to the love of his life rather than stealing him from the love of his life. In either case, such women are lying to themselves as much as to others involved.

Does it really matter if we fool strangers into believing something that isn't true? What harm is there in adapting little girl "dress up" as a fairy princess to adult-level social media in sharing fake or doctored photos as well as an invented name and background? Isn't pretending to be someone else on Facebook just another version of childhood pretend games? If so, the stakes for winning and losing are much higher for adults, with those caught using a false identity abandoned or, if used for illicit purposes such as a bank account, potentially receiving jail time or fines. So-called winners, on the other hand, may score a new relationship built on pretense that, like a house of cards, is poised to tumble at the least provocation. Many women fail to honestly appraise the situation.

With mounting cultural pressure on women to look eternally youthful and beautiful, it's no wonder that females of all ages feel driven to project an online persona that is nearly perfect and highly inaccurate. Women have been conditioned for centuries to believe that beauty is the basis for self-worth—at least in terms of competing for a husband. With a third of the current U.S. population at obese weight levels, women are struggling harder than ever to appear attractive by various means. Cosmetic surgery and an ever-growing range of beauty products feed the belief that no woman is beautiful in her own right; she must conform to either the "perfect" standard of beauty or others' impressions of feminine appeal, and thus, cover her true self with a façade of another person who is thinner, younger, and more attractive than the original version.

In accepting this cultural lie, women have been deceived and thus conditioned to become deceptive in who they are and what they really look like beneath the fake tan, fake nails, and fake hair. It's one thing to enhance a natural characteristic to look and feel better. But it's another to re-create an almost entirely new person that bears little resemblance to the original human being. Some women pay tens of thousands of dollars to modify every visible body part, from cheeks to nose to chin to breasts to tummy to buttocks. Do these women find themselves so distasteful that, like locusts, they discard their original "shell" and replace it with a veneer of self-improvement that transforms them into another person? Ironically, sculpting a new physical persona chips away at the inner person as well as the outer one.

Escaping a troubled past is a natural response to stress, shame, or failure. Some women who have been victimized by circumstances or other people forcibly try to forget their trauma and bury painful memories in their subconscious. Abuse, betrayal, and abandonment are just a few causes of extreme hurt that can cause some women to lie to themselves about the physical, emotional, or psychological damage they have sustained, and avoid treatment that could bring healing. Instead, the terrible experiences of the past rise up unexpectedly, like unbidden ghosts, to haunt them when they least expect it, eroding their self-esteem and peace of mind. Acknowledging hurt and seeking professional help are the first steps to self-honesty that can begin to restore emotional well-being.

DISHONESTY AND LOVED ONES

What about deceiving family members on noncritical issues? Is passing off a supermarket deli meatloaf as homemade as unethical as plagiarizing a colleague's publication for an upcoming presentation? Most people would say no, the meatloaf deception is not nearly as immoral as plagiarism. Using that logic, perhaps the decision depends on what is at stake. A meatloaf masquerade fools only friends or relatives, right? But a professional presentation impacts not only a career and reputation but also the representative company or organization.

Should a woman lie about her husband's problematic behavior? If he is too drunk to go to work, should she report him absent to keep from being fired? Substance abuse counselors would likely recommend that the wife should let her husband handle the consequences of his behavior rather than becoming enmeshed in his problem. But a wife that depends on her husband's income is highly motivated to help him keep his job so he can support the family. A heart-to-heart talk is important for the couple to begin addressing this critical issue, and professional help may be needed.

Similarly, what if a woman is being abused by her husband and covers it up to friends and relatives? Lying to protect her husband may likewise be in her self-interests. If he is prosecuted and goes to jail, she will lose a spouse and any income he brings to the household, and their children will lose a father. Women in these situations often lie to protect their husbands and boyfriends, as well as their own well-being, without realizing they may be making the problem worse by enabling the abuse to continue. Professional help may be necessary, and if the man won't go with her, the wife should consider going alone.

If a teenage son steals a piece of equipment from school, should the mother report it or keep quiet? Perhaps she doesn't want to get involved, or assumes her son will work through his guilt and do the right thing. If he is under the age of eighteen, however, she is responsible, and it is a parent's duty to make the child responsible, also. Actively lying, if called by the school, to say her son didn't steal the item or that she doesn't know if he did it is unethical. Some parents find it difficult to hold their children to moral standards. Just as important is the example that parents set by being actively or passively dishonest.

RELATIONAL HONESTY

Some women tend to be less than honest with their personal numbers—age, bodily measurements, weight, street address, and phone, for example. Numbers can be inflexible identifiers of information that ladies often prefer not to share, especially with those they don't know well. Numbers can't lie—at least not forever—so it is prudent to avoid their use when relevant facts should not be disclosed. This is often a safety feature of social networking interactions: share details that are not fixed, but only those that are moveable. As the maxim reminds us, it's hard to hit a moving target.

But once a relationship has formed, is it wise to play fast and loose with the truth? Which facts from prior experiences can and should be hidden? Do boyfriends and husbands need to know every detail about a woman's past? After all, what a person doesn't know can't hurt him, right?

It depends on what is considered to be critical knowledge. This will vary from one person to another. Some men don't care how many lovers a woman had before him. Other men want all the steamy details to ascertain their current position in a woman's life. How much information a woman chooses to reveal is quite individualized, and often depends on the nature of the relationship. In beginning a new dating relationship, many women feel no obligation to tell all their romantic secrets. Others, however, prefer to be straight-up honest with a new man in their lives. A woman may be prudent in avoiding a detailed account of her past for fear of upsetting her new beau. But if she is not emotionally invested, she may decide to be frank about her past and exchange personal histories with her new love interest. No precise social guidelines exist for this delicate process.

If she doesn't tell him everything up front, and if they get married, should she then spill the beans? Many couples choose to confess all prior relationships to each other when their present union deepens in intimacy. However, revealing too much information may give the partner a handy weapon to hurl when the couple ends up in a fight. For this reason some women decide to share only a brief account of their romantic history in a good-faith effort to be honest, while preserving the most private details in memory alone.

Uncertainties about honesty, especially pertaining to romantic and family relationships, include many issues, such as the wisdom of disclosing whether a couple got married before a child's birth, whether a child was adopted, and whether a couple practices mutual fidelity. Before questions arise, it is helpful to prepare answers that will suffice in various situations. School officials will probably need a different type and level of information than a neighbor, for example. Don't wait to be caught off-guard when it becomes easy and sometimes automatic to say something that isn't true.

What if a woman contracted a sexually transmitted disease (STD) that is in remission or treatable by monitoring symptoms, such as herpes simplex? Is she honor-bound to tell her new boyfriend, fiancé, or husband, or can she ethically keep this secret to herself if she believes there is little to no chance of his catching it? What if she is a victim of childhood abuse, has spent time in prison for a crime, or has been fired from a job for theft? Must she reveal all the sordid experiences of her past to the person with whom she is spending her life? In holding part of herself in reserve, what does a woman risk emotionally?

Living an inauthentic life also denies the possibility of feeling truly loved for who we are, and consequently we inevitably find ourselves caught in a relentless quest for love that can never be satisfied or sustained. How can I trust that anyone really loves me when I haven't shown who I really am? . . . . It's only when we both reveal ourselves fully that the deepest, purest, most soul-nourishing love can be exchanged. The remedy for engaging more fully is to first be in touch with what we are feeling and then to express, rather than repress, connect rather than protect, and reveal rather than conceal.

Although each of us chooses the degree of honesty that we will bestow on those who share our lives, it is important to weigh the pros and cons when making this important decision. Another way to approach the question is to consider how much of a partner's past a woman expects to be revealed? She can ask no more than she herself is willing to give.

Failing to reveal herself as a carrier of a potentially deadly STD such as AIDS or hepatitis C can have lethal consequences. The partner who unknowingly risks contracting a potentially fatal disease may pursue legal recourse on receiving a diagnosis tied to the female partner. A man who fathers children with a female disease carrier who has chosen not to reveal her condition may have children who inherit the disease—a choice he might not have knowingly made had the facts been stated. Even if the couple stays together, their relationship may be seriously damaged by withholding information of this type. Sometimes women are less likely to admit to having an STD for fear of reaping harsh punishment through criticism or rejection. Yet, the dangers of keeping such information secret can be even more damaging.

Another type of deception is to deny certain facts of their lives to prospective suitors for fear of losing them. Emma, a nurse, married a successful doctor with whom she had three children. Her husband became an alcoholic, routinely committed adultery, and eventually left her. Emma was devastated. For several years she hibernated, brooding on her losses. Then as her children grew up, she became lonely and opened herself to finding love again.

In her forties, Emma met a successful businessman. Fearing that he might also reject her one day, Emma set about systematically denying her age. Whenever the topic came up, she said she "wasn't sure" of her age because her parents had never told her specifically. Asked to see her driver's license, Emma claimed she had lost it and could not remember what birth date appeared on it. When it became known her new love interest had been hoping for a never-married woman, Emma insisted she had almost not been married at all because she and her husband didn't get along and he was gone much of the time. Emma's claims to youth and purity became so exaggerated and unbelievable that her beau's friends were hard-pressed not to tease her. The relationship did not last. Perhaps the moral of the story from this account is that in trying to reinvent our nature to attain a challenging goal, we may lose ourselves completely in the process.

Another form of deception is the outer veneer we put on in public, in contrast to the "real" person we are at home. Although most of us are different publicly and privately to some extent, the two selves seldom become totally distinct. A woman named Brenda, married to an associate pastor, appeared to be a typical social butterfly. Slender and energetic, she would buzz from one person to the next at church activities and celebrations, in a smiling and pleasant manner. But at home, she would take off the mask and complain to her husband about the congregational members they were supposed to minister to. Mrs. so-and-so was too heavy; Mr. so-and-so who talked too much. Not only did she gossip and criticize the innocent folks who assumed she was a kind and supportive person, but Brenda also encouraged a church member to divorce his wife when the couple began disputing finances, despite the fact that Brenda's church discouraged divorce except for serious reasons such as adultery or abuse. The man followed Brenda's advice and divorced his wife, leaving their two children floating between two households. The ex-wife became seriously depressed and was stuck with tens of thousands of dollars of the husband's accrued personal debt. None of this seemed to bother Brenda, who continued to display her public pious attitude.

Maintaining a dual personality generally leads to trouble. *A house divided cannot stand* is an old saying that still holds true.

When a problem arises with another person, it is best to go to that person directly and respectfully share any concerns. Asking questions instead of leveling accusations is a more productive way of dealing with issues. Sharing hurtful information with anyone else, except to seek clarity or request advice, is likely to rebound in destructive ways.

FLEXIBLE HONESTY

Flexible or careless honesty involves making light of the truth, twisting it in a variety of ways to suit momentary, transient needs. Although this is a characteristic evidenced in both sexes on occasion, in this book we are focusing on the woman.

Jane, a bubbly twenty-three-year-old college student, is a people pleaser. Neglected by her parents while growing up, she learned to say whatever would make someone happy—a caregiver, friend, romantic interest, teacher, whomever. Although Jane kept her dorm room temperature at seventy-five degrees, when a hometown girlfriend came to campus for a weekend visit and claimed the room seemed very warm, Jane quickly turned down the thermostat.

> "What temperature do you usually keep your room at?" the friend asked as she got under the covers of the futon. "I keep mine at sixty-eight; I can't bear being warm at night."

> "I always set mine at sixty-eight, too," Jane lied, her cheeks flushing pink.

A week later she told an aunt, her best friend, and a neighbor three versions of the same story about whether she would keep a stray kitten she'd found.

> "I'm going to keep it."

> "I might take it to the animal shelter."

> "I'm giving it to my sister back home."

Granted, Jane may have changed her mind about whether to keep the kitten, but she presented her decision as final to each of these three people, who inadvertently met at a birthday party shortly thereafter and unexpectedly discussed the story. It is possible that Jane may be a habitual liar, caused by childhood trauma or other unknown factors. She had been diagnosed with ADHD and took medicine for it sometimes but not consistently, which may have aggravated her confusion and impulsivity.

Although Jane's case may be unusual, it bears resemblance to those of women who casually mishandle the truth without guilt. Some don't view the truth as necessary. Consequently, they earn few people's trust. When confronted by those to whom they have been dishonest, women who lightly handle the truth make the following claims:

> "I forgot, but now I remember saying that."

"I might have said that."

"I didn't say that."

"I don't recall saying that at all."

Perhaps they don't remember, or maybe they don't want to admit being caught in a lie. It is advisable to avoid sharing confidential information with someone who cannot be trusted.

For many, truth is relative. For others, truth is absolute.

For all of us, honesty in personal or professional relationships is usually considered to be an important trait. Storytelling can be a fun pastime but should not be substituted for delivering the facts. The next time you are tempted to sidestep honesty, consider the consequences first. Sometimes complete honesty is unnecessary. At other times, it may be absolutely necessary. Learn to differentiate between situations where you will need to know the difference.

SUGGESTED STRATEGIES

1. If you occasionally practice commission of deceit or omission of truth, try to anticipate these situations before they occur. Then be honest about whatever information you plan to share. If you don't feel comfortable sharing anything, try to avoid the situation altogether or let others know you cannot participate.
2. Reflect on times when you tend to be dishonest with yourself. This can happen when you set unrealistic goals or downplay a weakness. Consider ways of more accurately or realistically describing the facts.
3. When a friend speaks vaguely, ask questions to help her be more specific and forthright. For example, if a roommate complains her boyfriend disrespects her, ask what that means or to give some examples. This will help her to carefully consider the impact of her complaint as well as support it with examples, or if not, revise her statement.
4. Speaking directly includes being honest, even when it can be difficult. Give some thought as to how you might approach a challenging topic that needs to be discussed with a friend or coworker.

REFERENCES

Bloom, Linda and Charlie Bloom. "The Cost and Benefits of Emotional Honesty." *Psychology Today* 12 Dec. 2011: n. pag. Web.
Ralston, Jeannie. "Lies In Marriage: What We Don't Tell Our Husbands." *Parenting* 1 Jan. 2012: n. pag. Web.

FOUR

Sense and Sensitivity

What role does emotion play in communication? Most of us express various emotions in many conversations. A few people reveal no emotion at all, maintaining a poker face. Some people interact with others through one main emotion, whereas others use a full spectrum of feelings to convey moods or opinions. People of all ages, including children, may be identified by a dominant emotional outlook: happy-go-lucky, sour, depressed. Conversely, those who display little or no emotion are frequently characterized as soulless, heartless, mindless, or lifeless, all of which convey a negative connotation.

The notions of emotions as a contributing factor to the communication process dates back many centuries. The ancient Greeks made much of emotion in their study of medicine as well as the arts. Their beliefs became the historical basis of primitive psychology and continued down through the medieval era and the Renaissance:

> The human body was thought to contain a mix of the four humors: black bile (also known as melancholy), yellow or red bile, blood, and phlegm. Each individual had a particular humoral makeup, or "constitution," and health was defined as the proper humoral balance for that individual. An imbalance of the humors resulted in disease.

The humors also referred to four individual psychological temperaments: melancholic, choleric, sanguine, and phlegmatic. This reflects the humoral concept that physical health and personality were part of the same whole.

The development of humoral theory is associated originally with Hippocrates (ca. 460–370 bce). In the second century CE, Galen elaborated on this theory, which was further developed by Arabic writers beginning in the ninth century and by European writers beginning in the eleventh. Though several important publications—including Andreas Vesalius's

De Humani Corporis Fabrica in 1543 and William Harvey's *De Motu Cordis* in 1628—challenged aspects of humoral theory, it remained dominant among physicians and the public through the nineteenth century.

Each humor was centered in a particular organ—brain, lung, spleen, and gall bladder—and related to a particular personality type—sanguine, phlegmatic, melancholic, and choleric. Though our understanding of psychology and emotions has continued to evolve, even today you may still hear someone say, "He's always in a good humor" or "She's in bad humor today"—a verbal throwback to previous beliefs.

In the twenty-first century, the study of emotion and its role in the human experience is complex. Psychologists, psychiatrists, counselors, physicians, and biologists explore the ways in which moods and feelings are transmitted through the body to become manifest outwardly to observers. Translating emotions as part of a communication exchange can have a vital impact on the meaning of a message. Perhaps that is why even technological communication (i.e., e-mail, texting, and Twitter) use lexicons that contain pictorial symbols called emoticons. Young people who frequently text make a point of adding "lol" or "ha ha" to downplay the seriousness of words typed in basic text code. All too often, however, in verbal or written exchanges, emotions can be misinterpreted, adding confusion to the conversation. Increasingly, specialists are consulted for help in learning how to use emotions correctly in communication.

The Occupational Outlook Handbook estimated that "Employment of psychologists is expected to grow 22 percent from 2010 to 2020, faster than the average for all occupations." Related professions are likewise expanding. This underscores the growing importance of psychology in postmodern culture, which includes the study of emotional implications of verbal and nonverbal communication. Improperly used or misunderstood, emotions can complicate meaning.

In certain occupations, emotional displays are discouraged if not downright forbidden: modeling is one example. The goal is to get viewers to focus on the fashions being strutted on the stage or displayed in an advertisement, not get fixated on the beautiful model. In the acting field, however, the opposite is true, with actors depicting different emotions based on the role being played. Those employed in professional occupations, such as lawyers, doctors, and teachers, typically limit emotions in their interactions. Although they are likely to show certain emotions on occasion, such as humor or anger, they are expected to maintain a professional façade of courtesy and emotional detachment from clients, patients, or students. Generally, emotion is kept on a tight rein in the professions.

So when is it appropriate to display personal emotions in conversation? Should all feelings be repressed except in the company of close friends and relatives? Some cultures represent emotions in differing ways, but in the United States, we are fairly open to sharing emotions as long as we don't overdo it. Too little or too much can negatively impact a conversation.

There are times when just basic information is desired, especially in a business exchange, and thus many companies use telephone recordings and on-hold messages to inform callers of relevant facts. But many people prefer to interact with living, breathing humans who are willing to exchange emotions in small talk or a funny story while doing business. What would it be like to go grocery shopping without a casual exchange of pleasantries at the checkout counter? Of course, self-checkout is growing in popularity to save the business world money and customers time. Many commercial transactions are going the technological route amid debates about the value of a human face and voice. Rapidly disappearing are polite civilities, spontaneous questions, holiday greetings, and shared jokes as robots and machines replace human workers. Should we completely exclude emotional expressions—verbal or nonverbal—from professional interactions?

At the University of Michigan Health Systems Employee Assistance Program, Jeanne Segal and colleagues have posted an informational site called "Emotion Communicates! The powerful role emotions play in all relationships" as a resource for the campus and the community:

> When you are aware and in control of your emotions, you can think clearly and creatively; manage stress and challenges; communicate well with others; and display trust, empathy, and confidence. But lose control of your emotions, and you'll spin into confusion, isolation, and doubt. By learning to recognize, manage, and deal with your emotions, you'll enjoy greater happiness and health, as well as better relationships.

Thus, emotion that is honestly acknowledged and appropriately managed can enhance rather than disrupt communication.

In fact, an entire scientific area of research has evolved from the study of emotions, and specifically, emotional intelligence. Daniel Goleman, author of bestselling book *Emotional Intelligence: Why It Can Matter More than IQ*, explains on his Website how the growing understanding of emotional intelligence has filtered through our society to permeate countless areas, from entertainment to education:

> the concept has been embraced by educators, in the form of programs in social and emotional learning or SEL . . . tens of thousands of schools worldwide offer children SEL. In the United States many districts and even entire states currently make SEL curriculum requirement, mandating that just as students must attain a certain level of competence in math and language, so too should they master these essential skills for living. . . .
>
> The data show that SEL programs yielded a strong benefit in academic accomplishment, as demonstrated in achievement test results and grade-point averages. In participating schools, up to 50 percent of

children showed improved achievement scores and up to 38 percent improved their grade-point averages. SEL programs also made schools safer: incidents of misbehavior dropped by an average of 28 percent; suspensions by 44 percent; and other disciplinary actions by 27 percent. At the same time, attendance rates rose, while 63 percent of students demonstrated significantly more positive behavior. . . .

Perhaps the biggest surprise for me has been the impact of EI in the world of business, particularly in the areas of leadership and employee development (a form of adult education). *The Harvard Business Review* has hailed emotional intelligence as "a ground-breaking, paradigm-shattering idea," one of the most influential business ideas of the decade.

As Goleman indicates, emotional intelligence is a valuable human commodity that can serve us well in personal or professional contexts. However, it must be clearly understood to become fully useful.

Goleman's research spawned an explosion of discoveries and resources dedicated to the dissemination of information about emotional intelligence. One such resource, the Consortium for Research on Emotional Intelligence in Organizations, comprises ten core members and seventy-eight individual members with track records in applied research. The Website offers article reprints, model programs, and references, among other things, to inform interested readers about the nature of this social behavior.

Social awareness refers to how people handle interpersonal relationships and awareness of others' feelings, needs, and concerns. Related organizational behaviors include influence, as in wielding effective tactics for persuasion, and conflict management—negotiating and resolving disagreements. Learning to become more sensitive to other people can lead to more direct interactions and meaningful communication.

Working with a counselor or psychologist, anyone can be tested on emotional intelligence using the most applicable instrument for their needs. There are numerous tests and questionnaires that can be completed to reveal a person's emotional intelligence level, including personal strengths and weaknesses.

Let's look at some ways that emotions can impact a friendship or a relationship. For example, if you have a friend with a knack for pushing all your wrong buttons, there's a good chance you are often at odds with each other. Although conflict can be healthy in helping people come to terms with their differences, it can also be harmful if left unresolved or allowed to escalate. How can this tendency impact the honesty or directness of your interpersonal communication?

Untamed emotions can invade a pleasant conversation and turn it into a verbal free-for-all, with one or both parties hurling "truths" at the other without thought to consequences:

"You always make everything about you! I'm sick of it!"

"And I hate that color on you, by the way!"

"Everyone says you're a jerk!"

True or not, statements like these have a damaging impact, especially when spoken in the heat of anger. If such things must be said, it's better to wait for the right time, when both people are calm, and then to say them in a purposeful way with the intent of helping, not hurting, the other person.

In the business world, being frank is usually a valued trait, preferably without the innuendo of emotion. Sighs, eye-rolling, and headshakes can be helpful body language in conjunction with dialogue. But when exaggerated, they suggest a hostile attitude that may interfere with positive interaction.

Emotions should never be ignored. But they need to be harnessed and work in tandem with other communication skills. For example, if you are angry because the raise you received at work is less than you expected, you don't have to slough it off. You may have good reasons to go to the appropriate administrator to discuss your concern. However, it is far better to express your disappointment politely ("I was surprised to get just a 2 percent raise") than to rush into someone's office, yelling profanities and threats.

Acknowledging your emotions is an important part of communicating honestly with yourself. Sharing your emotions is likewise critical in telling others how you feel. Just be sure to express feelings in a productive way, respectfully, in a constrained manner. Displays of temper or distress can do more harm than good and keep the other person's attention off the source of the problem (i.e., a disappointing raise, a denial of a vacation request, or the mandate to work Saturdays). When we force others to put out emotional fires, they probably have few resources (and perhaps little patience) left for dealing with core issues.

Similarly, in personal relationships, it is critical to be honest. It just doesn't pay to hide or ignore emotions over things that matter. There are plenty of nonessential issues that annoy us, probably daily. If they do not impact our values or principles we might do well to sputter and fume in private, where our emotions cannot harm or alarm others.

In major dilemmas that spike emotions, we must learn to recognize our reactions and control sharp feelings before speaking. Dzogchen Ponlop Rinpoche, author of *Rebel Buddha*, discusses the out-of-control sense that often accompanies strong emotions:

> Once emotion bursts out and overflows, all bets are off. We get caught in its momentum and abandon all reason. We may often say or do things we'll regret, so we end up fearful of our emotions. If we feel

anger rising up toward our partner, for example, we might panic and try to shut it down or get rid of it. In that case, we might turn the anger in on ourselves or let it loose on an innocent target—a co-worker, a child, or the family pet. Or we might be successful in keeping our angry mind quiet for a few weeks, then blow up one day for no apparent reason. When it's over we're exhausted, but not necessarily any clearer about what happened or why. Because there's no real resolution, the seeds are planted for a repeat performance.

Have you ever been told something that made your blood boil? That is not the time to lash out at the other person. If you do speak up, it is likely you will say things you will regret later. Being told by the doctor that you need to lose weight may not be what you want to hear, especially if your schedule is already busy with limited time for meal planning and exercise. Instead of angrily telling the doctor that she has no clue how hard it is for you to add one more thing to your daily routine, give yourself time to think about it. Then, if you must respond, do so politely, just as you would like to be addressed if the roles were reversed.

Sometimes a person will use "honesty" in a passive-aggressive way to repel an annoying acquaintance. One of the ways this can be done is by bringing up a sore subject to the other person. If you know he doesn't like religion, you might "accidentally" forget and begin discussing it. Or if a coworker becomes anxious around a certain administrator, you might mention that the administrator may be stopping by later, which could very well be a truthful fact, but one you only mention to "scare off" your annoying colleague so she'll return to her desk and stop bothering you.

Some people use emotions to convey a specific impression. For example, a prevalent social stereotype is that women who are pulled over by police officers for traffic violations often resort to tears to play on an officer's sympathy, especially a male officer. Surprisingly, it works rather well, and many get off the hook. Some women break into tears when an argument with a significant other becomes heated. Because men are often uneasy around crying women, some readily back off, conceding victory.

Another emotional "type" is the joker, who makes a jest of everything, often using harsh verbal barbs dressed as witticisms to poke fun at oth-

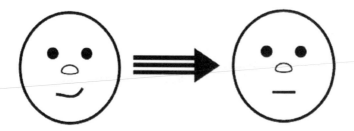

Figure 4.1.   Sensitivity and multi-faceted communication

ers, saying "I was just kidding" or "I didn't mean it." Because much of what she says is true and perhaps a thinly disguised effort to be straightforward, the effort fails, either in being received as a misguided joke or in hurting the hearer's feelings.

Then there is the bully, with a belligerent attitude who takes out her anger on others. Cloaked in the armor of self-righteousness, she attacks victims without warning and sometimes without cause to give them a piece of her mind. Because she is used to having her say and getting her way, little can be done to stop her tirade once it begins. Often it is best to simply avoid her. If you are unfairly attacked, maintain a normal voice level and calmly ask the person to explain the problem so that you can work on it; refuse to be drawn into needless conflict. As much as possible, try to work toward a win–win solution. If that is not possible, be prepared to confront the person in a reasonable way to defend yourself and rebuff undue criticism.

Someone with a woe-is-me attitude who expects you to join the pity party should be encouraged to become proactive. Sometimes there are no easy answers to life's problems, and we just have to "grin and bear it." A gentle reminder is often helpful. Those that try to unload too much of their personal life in the name of honesty may be leaning more toward confession. If it gets to the point where you feel uncomfortable, urge the person to contact a counselor for professional assistance.

The unemotional partner in a personal relationship can drive the other person crazy—not from expressing too much emotion, or the wrong kind, but from failure to display any kind of emotional response, especially during conflict. The other partner may wrongly interpret a lack of emotion as an uncaring attitude.

In all likelihood, the calm person may be experiencing similar emotions as the more outspoken partner, except not to the same degree, and certainly not demonstrated in the same way. She may feel inadequate in showing the expected feelings or fear losing control once she begins to open up emotionally. In cases such as these it can be helpful for the more reserved person to say something like this: "I feel angry too, but let's try to keep the problem in perspective and decide what to do."

On the other end of the emotional spectrum are those who cannot bear to hear the truth, no matter how gently or prudently it is presented. A teenager whose boyfriend tells her he does not want to be exclusive may become hysterical at being rejected, disregarding the boyfriend's sound logic and admirable honesty. The woman who begs her husband to be truthful and admit he finds another woman attractive may subject him to a full emotional tirade when he does so, although he has not acted on his attraction. Requesting honesty on the grounds of relationship integrity can be a tenuous process. Honesty should not be punished by fury or desolation. Sincere honesty should be met with a self-controlled response that leads to meaningful dialogue. It is best not to ask for truth until you are prepared to deal with it responsibly.

Emotions are another handy resource to add to the communication tool belt. When assessed honestly and shared openly, with decorum and practicality, personal feelings add a rich dimension to any relationship. Applied incorrectly, they can do more harm than good. Like a builder's screwdriver or hammer, emotions should be handled with skill for constructive purposes and should be carefully labeled and appropriately used for a productive outcome.

SUGGESTED STRATEGIES

1. If you are aware of an upcoming discussion where you could get emotional, you might want to postpone the meeting until you have had a chance to process your feelings. Try to understand why you feel as you do, and then decide how to channel your emotions appropriately.
2. When you are having a conversation in which you become strongly emotional, ask for a timeout of perhaps a few minutes to pull yourself together. If you need more time, postpone the conversation.
3. As emotions surface in communication, it helps to be aware of their source. Understanding that you feel sad on Christmas Eve each year because that's when your mother passed away decades before will help you deal with your feelings and plan holiday events accordingly.
4. Get to know your emotional triggers. If certain topics make you feel angry or frustrated, avoid them in conversation. When they must be addressed, understand how your emotions are in play rather than letting them control you.

REFERENCES

Goleman, Daniel. "Emotional Intelligence." N.p., n.d. Web. 16 Dec. 2013. http://www.danielgoleman.info/topics/emotional-intelligence.

"Humoral Theory." Contagion: Historical Views of Diseases and Epidemics, Harvard University, n.d. Web. 16 Dec. 2013. http://ocp.hul.harvard.edu/contagion/humoral-theory.html.

"Psychologists." Occupational Outlook Handbook, United States Department of Labor, n.d. Web. 16 Dec. 2013. http://www.bls.gov/ooh/Life-Physical-and-Social-Science/Psychologists.htm.

Rinpoche, Dzogchen Ponlop. "Relationships: Riding Your Emotional Rollercoaster." *Huffington Post* 7 July 2010, sec. Lifestyle: n. pag. Print.

Segal, Jeanne, Melinda Smith, and Lawrence Robinson. "Emotion Communicates! The powerful role emotions play in all relationships." UMHS EAP, n.d. Web. 13 Dec. 2013. http://www.sitemaker.umich.edu/um-aaop/files/emotion_communicates.pdf.

FIVE

His Fault/Her Fault

It Started in Eden

We've all heard the story: In the legendary garden, a beautiful and be-guiling serpent persuades Eve to eat forbidden fruit—to counter God's only prohibition to her and husband Adam.

Perhaps exulting in and expanding her independent nature, Eve not only eats the forbidden fruit but she also convinces Adam to indulge, which seals their fate of bringing God's curses on them and their descen-dents and exiling them from the perfect garden paradise.

Adam and Eve's disobedience led to their expulsion from the Garden and the legacy of gender-based curses that continue down to the present. Women were condemned to experience great pain in childbirth and sus-tain a strong desire for a husband, whereas men would endure harsh physical labor. Whether you consider the story literal truth or symbolic myth, the saga of Adam and Eve continues to influence our world today. Throughout literary history and Judeo-Christian doctrine, the story re-sounds as a lesson in human frailty. The actual characters are referenced in the Bible and surface periodically in literature through works such as John Milton's *Paradise Lost* (1667). Early American fiction makes frequent use of the Adam and Eve motif, with Puritan figures such as Nathaniel Hawthorne's "Young Goodman Brown" reenacting humanity's fall from grace. Joni Mitchell's song about the 1969 Woodstock Festival includes a veiled reference to the "garden" to suggest a back-to-nature motif and fresh start for contemporary youth. In today's entertainment industry, Adam and Eve would be rock stars.

Although the account found in Genesis 3 of the Bible has inspired countless retellings and interpretations, few have examined the commu-nication implications. Throughout history, communication between men and women has always been haphazard at best and perhaps began that way in the very first union. If only Adam and Eve had been clear with each other. . . .

Let's take a closer look at what happened. Reviewing the details of those fateful events offers insight to husband-and-wife communication and the question of direct vs. indirect speech. Here is the story as given in Genesis 3 (*New American Standard* version):

> Now the serpent was more crafty than any beast of the field which the Lord God had made. And he said to the woman, "Indeed, has God said, 'You shall not eat from any tree of the garden'?" ² The woman said to the serpent, "From the fruit of the trees of the garden we may eat; ³ but from the fruit of the tree which is in the middle of the garden, God has said, 'You shall not eat from it or touch it, or you will die.'" ⁴ The serpent said to the woman, "You surely will not die! ⁵ For God knows that in the day you eat from it your eyes will be opened, and you will be like God, knowing good and evil." ⁶ When the woman saw that the tree was good for food, and that it was a delight to the eyes, and that the tree was desirable to make *one* wise, she took from its fruit and ate; and she gave also to her husband with her, and he ate. ⁷ Then the eyes of both of them were opened, and they knew that they were naked; and they sewed fig leaves together and made themselves loin coverings.
>
> ⁸ They heard the sound of the Lord God walking in the garden in the cool of the day, and the man and his wife hid themselves from the presence of the Lord God among the trees of the garden. ⁹ Then the Lord God called to the man, and said to him, "Where are you?" ¹⁰ He said, "I heard the sound of You in the garden, and I was afraid because I was naked; so I hid myself." ¹¹ And He said, "Who told you that you were naked? Have you eaten from the tree of which I commanded you not to eat?" ¹² The man said, "The woman whom You gave *to be* with me, she gave me from the tree, and I ate." ¹³ Then the Lord God said to the woman, "What is this you have done?" And the woman said, "The serpent deceived me, and I ate." ¹⁴ The Lord God said to the serpent,
>
> "Because you have done this, Cursed are you more than all cattle, And more than every beast of the field; On your belly you will go, And dust you will eat All the days of your life; ¹⁵ And I will put enmity Between you and the woman, And between your seed and her seed; He shall bruise you on the head, And you shall bruise him on the heel."
>
> ¹⁶ To the woman He said, "I will greatly multiply Your pain in childbirth, In pain you will bring forth children; Yet your desire will be for your husband, And he will rule over you."
>
> ¹⁷ Then to Adam He said, "Because you have listened to the voice of your wife, and have eaten from the tree about which I commanded you, saying, 'You shall not eat from it';
>
> Cursed is the ground because of you; In toil you will eat of it All the days of your life. ¹⁸ "Both thorns and thistles it shall grow for you; And you will eat the plants of the field; ¹⁹ By the sweat of your face You will

eat bread, Till you return to the ground, Because from it you were taken; For you are dust, And to dust you shall return."

The three individuals in this drama personify the eternal triangle, albeit a spiritual rather than a sexual one. God presides over the series of events, from the creation of the garden and its inhabitants to the humans' punishment and exile. Stated and implied conversations, along with narration, tell what happened and reveal the nature of each speaker.

Adam and Eve appear to be a contented young couple in a stress-free environment; at least we are given no indication otherwise.

Enter the smooth-talking serpent. He approaches Eve, perhaps sensing a more vulnerable victim than Adam, and he questions her in depth about the one rule she and Adam were expected to follow: they could eat anything in the garden, except from tree of knowledge of good and evil, which was centrally located where it would be a continual reminder and temptation.

In this translation, the serpent prefaces his question with "Indeed," suggesting that he is responding to Eve's prior statement. Their conversation may have started long before this particular question is raised.

"Indeed, has God said, 'You shall not eat from any tree of the garden'?"

To this basic fourteen-word question, Eve responds in forty-three words—more than three times as many. Evidently she is drawn in by the trick question, feeling the need to provide an adequate defense and correct the serpent's understanding.

In turn, the serpent refutes God's admonition: "[4] The serpent said to the woman, "You surely will not die! [5] For God knows that in the day you eat from it your eyes will be opened, and you will be like God, knowing good and evil."

Disarmed, Eve concedes the battle of words and obedience to the stranger and accepts the forbidden fruit. Moreover, she shares it with Adam, who apparently is right beside her. Was Adam a voyeur watching a stranger seduce his wife?

> [6] When the woman saw that the tree was good for food, and that it was a delight to the eyes, and that the tree was desirable to make *one* wise, she took from its fruit and ate; and she gave also to her husband *with her*, and he ate. [emphasis mine]

Surrendering her allegiance to God and husband, Eve admires the fruit on several levels—taste, beauty, and wisdom—and willingly takes it from the tree to share with Adam. Interestingly, there is no record that Adam protests or tries to dissuade her. In fact, he appears to completely support her disobedience, tacitly if not actively, and becomes complicit in her rebellion.

Was Eve enticed by the fruit or by the stranger's seductive nature? Was she convinced by his argument against God's prohibition—a cosmic powerplay that made her heady by inclusion as the one human player in the supernatural tug-of-war? Was the first female already trying to break through the glass ceiling of a male-dominated universe?

What we have learned since then is that several language studies support the idea that women typically speak more words than men, although some communication experts such as Deborah Tannen refute this claim. It is not absolutely true in all men or women, but it is fairly common and well documented. In a book titled *The Female Mind* discussed in the UK *Mail Online*, Dr Luan Brizendine claims that women's bodies devote more brain cells to talking than men. "The simple act of talking triggers a flood of brain chemicals which give women a rush similar to that felt by heroin addicts when they get a high." Think about it: in a couple that you know, which gender spends more time communicating by phone, text, social media, or e-mail? For many women, communication is a fun pastime as well as a necessary outlet. Men do not seem to use communication for the same reasons or to a similar degree.

Medical research continues to explore biological explanations for this phenomenon, as indicated in a recent study led by psychologist J. Michael Bowers and neuroscientist Margaret McCarthy:

> Despite recent progress toward sexual equality, it's still a man's world in many ways. But numerous studies show that when it comes to language, girls start off with better skills than boys. Now, scientists studying a gene linked to the evolution of vocalizations and language have for the first time found clear sex differences in its activity in both rodents and humans, with the gene making more of its protein in girls. But some researchers caution against drawing too many conclusions about the gene's role in human and animal communication from this study.
>
> Back in 2001, . . . a gene called *FOXP2* appeared to be essential for the production of speech. . . .
>
> During this same time period, a number of studies have confirmed past research suggesting that young girls learn language faster and earlier than boys, producing their first words and sentences sooner and accumulating larger vocabularies faster. But the reasons behind such findings are highly controversial because it is difficult to separate the effects of nature versus nurture, and the differences gradually disappear as children get older.

Studies such as these raise interesting questions. Was Eve better equipped to communicate than Adam, explaining why the serpent chose to approach her instead of him? Maybe Adam was the quiet type or preoccupied. If Eve felt neglected, she would have been flattered by the stranger's attention, by his conversation, by his willingness to enlighten her to the "truth" about the fruit, and by appearing to be the more correct or at least the more proximate supernatural figure with whom she could dialogue while God is temporarily out of the picture.

Emboldened by the stranger's interest, Eve takes the initiative and becomes the ringleader of the couple's rebellious escapade. As stated in Genesis 1:26–28, the couple had been created as equals to rule jointly over creation:

> [27] God created man in His own image, in the image of God He created him; male and female He created them. [28] God blessed them; and God said to them, "Be fruitful and multiply, and fill the earth, and subdue it; and rule over the fish of the sea and over the birds of the sky and over every living thing that moves on the earth."

Now Eve adopts an authoritative role in the relationship. She notes that the fruit is suitable to eat, attractive to admire, and desirable for wisdom; perhaps eating it would make her and Adam as wise as the serpent. She must have felt highly flattered. The creature had singled out her, not Adam. There may have been a touch of smugness in Eve's attitude when she offered the fruit to Adam, who readily ate it. Clearly, this was one of those times when the couple should have had a detailed discussion about the implications of giving in to temptation before seeking instant gratification. Any words exchanged with Adam, however, are not reported in the account. If he was the strong, silent type, maybe Eve just handed him the fruit and he took it without a word. In this pivotal passage, it is interesting that there is no indication that language of any type passed between the couple, suggesting potential conversation was nonexistent or unimportant, when its absence may have made a huge difference in the outcome of this story and the unfolding of human history.

It was only after God confronted the pair in their newfound knowledge of "nakedness" — physical and spiritual — that their communication styles change. They quickly blame each other rather than accept personal responsibility. Finally we hear Adam speak: "[12] The man said, 'The woman whom You gave *to be* with me, she gave me from the tree, and I ate.'" Adam appears to blame both God and Eve to exonerate himself. Interestingly, Adam now uses nearly three times as many words as Eve (nineteen versus seven), abandoning his masculine stance to adopt his wife's feminine communication style, whereas Eve assumes the masculine persona of uttering almost one-third fewer words than her husband, possibly underscoring their exchange of original gender roles:

> [13] Then the Lord God said to the woman, "What is this you have done?"
> And the woman said, "The serpent deceived me, and I ate."

Why the identity switch in terms of language? The couple's disobedience and deception led to confused gender roles that God will now forcefully address. Adam failed to protect his wife from the stranger's advances, and Eve neglected to discuss the stranger's temptation with her husband. God seems to hold Adam more responsible in pronouncing work-related consequences to him in seventy-two words, whereas Eve's curse based on domestic roles of wife and mother requires just thirty-one words, less than half the sum used for Adam.

Let's examine communication problems that led to the deadly deed.

First, Eve was seduced into confiding in a stranger. Tradition suggests the serpent was beautiful, perhaps adorned in bold colors and glittery scales. Certainly the fact that a snake could speak was wondrous enough. Eve fell for his lies—as all too often we do when confronted by temptations from shadowy sources.

Next, Eve disregarded the central authority to which she was responsible. Instead of going to God with questions or consulting her husband, she and Adam unilaterally countered God's command with the decision to disobey.

Then Eve shared her mistake with her husband. Apparently she phrased the temptation in such a way that he did not question her, just as she had not questioned the serpent. Adam accepted the fruit and ate it. Eve could have asked Adam's opinion, or they could have debated the pros and cons. But no conversation is recorded—a total lack of direct communication.

When their disobedience was discovered, Eve dodged responsibility while pointing to the serpent. Although it's true the creature did beguile her, it was Eve's decision to fall under his influence. She fails to honestly confess and repent. There does not appear to be any effort to apologize. Eve simply shifted blame and refused to be held accountable for her actions, as did Adam.

Thus, Eve failed to communicate effectively with three key persons in this story:

1. She should have challenged the serpent's credentials and sought God's clarification.
2. She should have honored her commitment instead of compromising her values.
3. She should have discussed the issue with Adam.
4. She should have admitted her failings and apologized.

Adam likewise made several communication blunders:

1. He passively failed to protect his wife from the stranger's advances.
2. He morally failed to encourage Eve and himself to remain obedient.
3. He completely failed to dissuade Eve from eating the fruit, and shared it with her.
4. He fearfully hid from God and passed blame.

Direct communication could have changed the course of literal or mythical history. Eve exercised her communication skills by using them for self-centered purposes. Far from questioning her, Adam went along with her plan. Neither appears to have spoken directly to the other about the temptation or its consequences, which was a life-changing and history-making event.

PASS THE BLAME, PLEASE

When you think of couples that are having problems, how many accept responsibility for their share of conflict? To put it another way, how many are pointing exclusively at the spouse or partner as the trouble source? Of those that do so, have they tried addressing the problem directly in a calm and rational discussion? Some spouses make little effort to truly understand the complexities of relationship conflict, much less their loved one's perspective. If they would explain their feelings without blaming the other person, progress might be made.

A contributing factor is that today, people often hook up or marry for self-gratification. They choose partners who are attractive, accomplished, or wealthy on the basis of how those assets will benefit them. They put far less time into considering how they can enrich the partner's life or the sacrifices that will be necessary to make the relationship work. Commitment and marriage are not the ideal environment for single-minded advancement. Rather, they offer the perfect framework for team effort. Those who are seeking personal gratification may prefer to stay single until that mindset changes because healthy relationships require clear communication.

In the past, most societies were rural, meaning that community members and marriage partners relied on each other for survival. Families tended to be large with numerous children because perhaps one-third to half died before reaching adulthood prior to a time when widespread health practices evolved. A man would choose a fertile wife (as suggested by a curvaceous figure or numerous siblings) to produce several healthy children. Women, on the other hand—when they could choose a husband as opposed to having one chosen for them—frequently selected a man of

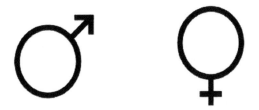

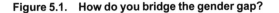

Figure 5.1.   How do you bridge the gender gap?

means, one who would economically support them and the resulting offspring.

Over time, as rural societies became industrialized, farm life was replaced by an urban lifestyle. Farmers became factory workers, with coins rather than cucumbers taken to market. Farmwives transitioned into housewives with new machines to assist with domestic chores, giving them more time to shop with their husbands' income.

Never before in history had so many women been given access to so many financial resources. More women managed a growing household income (eventually their own earnings as well as their husband's when women began entering the workforce). A husband's income level and his wife's household management sometimes led to sharp quarrels, especially as in many couples, one tends to be a spender and the other a saver. To escape rising tensions, some spouses avoided the home front to pursue other interests, such as gambling, drinking, or having an affair.

Today, many marriage experts agree that changing incentives in society, along with a shift in the balance of domestic power, helps to fuel irritations and frustrations that can lead to marital conflicts. Becoming less interdependent and more independent in marriage can be healthy, but those who pull too far apart may experience relational problems, as communication dwindles into monosyllabic exchanges or polite but meaningless conversation. When serious conflicts arise, spouses typically accuse each other rather than accept personal responsibility. Blame gets bandied back and forth like a tennis ball until one partner "wins," often at the expense of relational damage.

SHIFTING RELATIONSHIP PATTERNS

Nowadays, more spouses are maintaining separate households because of the rising number of long-distance marriages. This may be one reason why marriage is falling out of favor with youth, many of whom are instead opting to live together or have a family with a sperm or egg donor. The traditional family structure is dissolving and re-forming into new configurations that must be factored into the social equation, which makes communication even more challenging.

Let's say a thirty-year-old woman has two sons by different men. One man she has not seen in years; nor does he see his son. The other man comes and goes randomly, depending on the good nature of a third man the mother is currently seeing. If the absentee father should reappear, think of the potential for confusion when these four individuals—six if you count the two boys—try to communicate with each other. With emotions and allegiances in a continual state of flux, it will likely be difficult for these people to be open and direct with each other. Yet, for the sake of the children, anything less than clear communication could have a detrimental impact on the loosely related individuals.

Similarly, in households with stepchildren, it is frequently difficult for the nonbiological parent to communicate directly with a stepchild for fear of reprisal from the biological parent or because of emotional detachment from the child. Again, the situation depends on personality and relationship status, but the growing number of nontraditional family structures has led to indirect communication in many families. Efforts to have conflict-free conversations often escalate into powder kegs of emotion that can instantly explode when lit by an inflammatory word.

For example, ten-year-old Elena lives with her mother and the mother's boyfriend on weekdays, and with her biological father (who did not marry her mother) on weekends. Elena often hears both biological parents speak to their respective friends and family members about the other parent. Although cautioned not to repeat the things she overhears, Elena sometimes forgets and says something she should not and then hastily asks the parent she has spoken to not to tell the other parent. Of course, this can happen in a traditional family as well. But in a complicated situation with a diverse range of parental partners moving through a child's life, it is difficult for the child to speak openly to either parent consistently, and it is challenging for biological parents to have meaningful discussions about the child with several stepparents involved.

When Elena's paternal grandmother invited Elena and her mother to a Christmas concert, Elena happily said they would come, and she would relay the invitation to her mother. The grandmother bought tickets for Elena and her mom, only to discover two days before the concert that Elena had forgotten to ask her mom about the concert. As a result, Elena was able to go after some last-minute rescheduling by her mother, but her grandmother was out the $17.50 ticket purchased for the mom, who had scheduled other plans with her live-in boyfriend. It's not unusual for kids to forget to share a message, but asking a child to serve as messenger among several households is tricky.

BUSINESS COMMUNICATION

In the business world, men often prefer linear communication and brief discourse. Women, however, frequently use indirect speech and more detailed interactions.

In an article titled "High Octane Women," Sherrie Bourg Carter explains her perspective on direct versus indirect styles of communication:

> **Direct versus Indirect:** When you need something done, there are two basic ways you can communicate that need: directly or indirectly. Some people are very direct. When they want, need, or feel something, they come right out and say it. For example, "I want to move closer to the

kids' school." That's pretty direct; therefore, there is little room for misunderstanding what the speaker is saying. There are others, however, who prefer to test the waters before jumping in head first. They don't immediately (or in some extreme cases, ever) say exactly what they want, need, or feel. Examples of indirect communication are: "The school is pretty far from the house," or something a little less indirect like, "I wish we lived a little closer to the school." . . .

Your partner might get the sense that you'd like to move closer, but could just as easily miss the underlying message altogether. The latter statement isn't as vague, but it's not a direct statement either. Depending on the situation, we all use both direct and indirect forms of communication, but most people lean toward one style or another.

When people use direct communication, there is less risk for misunderstanding, yet more risk for offending or surprising the "receiver" by the directness of the message. With indirect communication, there is more risk for misunderstanding but less risk of offending the "receiver." In either case, when the two different styles come together in conversation, there is a greater likelihood for tension and stress in the relationship.

EMOTIONS VERSUS LOGIC

In recent years many spouses have adopted a touchy-feely approach to communication. Marriage manuals recommend tackling issues via emotions rather than by logic:

"When you come home late without calling, I *feel* disrespected."

But should a spouse take responsibility for your feelings rather than his behavior?

Many people shrink from speaking their minds. Instead, they try to say things that won't offend the hearer, taking responsibility for negative feelings rather than expecting the listener to accept responsibility for negative actions. It's not surprising that communication today is more confusing than ever.

If a woman says to her mate, "Please call when you are going to be late" instead of "I feel unimportant when you don't tell me you'll be late," her significant other can choose to comply with or ignore her request. If details are needed, like "why" he should inform her he'll be late, she can ask. Although it is important to share feelings with loved ones, emotions do not necessarily have to become the basis for every request or the pretext for an argument.

Research over the past several years indicates men's tendency toward direct communication and women's toward an indirect approach, as supported by the findings of Vinita Mohindra and Samina Azhar:

> Men's and women's differing communication styles are based both in
> science and nature. As the ancient hunters and gatherers, men were
> often put into a position of competition. They were competing against
> nature while trying to hunt and capture dinner. They were competing
> against one another for tribal status and mates. Winning, whether in a
> fight against an animal or a fellow tribesman, meant staying alive.
> Women, on the other hand, were often put into a position of coopera-
> tion as the family caretakers. They would band together to help with
> child care and other domestic duties. For women, avoiding fights
> meant staying alive. That history still affects us today. Men are compet-
> itive and hierarchical. They establish rank and status. Women look for
> similarities and value cooperation. In conclusion, no matter what com-
> munication style is adopted both men and women will communicate in
> different ways. Men will take the approach of instrumental communi-
> cation style where they want the answer right away and establish their
> hierarchy and supremacy. Women, on the other hand, will be more of
> an expressive style of communication as they will be able to confide in
> others and are more sensitive to issues than men women will be able to
> build, maintain and strengthen the relationship. (27)

Although it is essential to speak carefully and with consideration for
the hearer, it is just as important to be honest and forthright about the
speaker's concerns. Of course, any heartfelt discussion can escalate into a
full-blown argument, so that both parties say exactly what they think—in
extreme detail—without thought for possible repercussions. That type of
honesty does not usually render productive results. The overarching goal
should be sincere self-expression that is helpful rather than hurtful.

IMPRESSIONS OF UNCERTAINTY

Women who speak indirectly not only sometimes fail to clearly communicate the desired message but they also may be perceived as inadequate
or unfocused, particularly in professional settings. In some cases, a ques-
tionable image may negatively impact their career. How do others who
scarcely know a particular woman interpret her communication style as
indirect? Monica Hersh Khetarpal Sholar discusses typical conventions
by indicating that women's indirect speech "contains many hedges" such
as "sorta" and "y'know" along with tag questions such as "this room is
warm, isn't it?" instead of making a clear statement: "This room is
warm."

Furthermore, using intensifiers such as "so" and "such" as well as a
weak tone of voice are characteristic of indirect speech (92). To these
traits Sholar adds that women are likelier than men to use plural first-
person pronouns such as "we" and "us" and are less likely to make
emphatic statements, such as "She lied," and instead say something like
"She wasn't honest" or "She evidently didn't tell the truth." Several re-

searchers claim that men make more statements based on logic, whereas women tend to speak from personal experience or observation. Again, this is not always the case.

Some women use plentiful detail when they speak, which other women often appreciate, whereas some men may not. The latter may tune out a woman who includes significant description in her narratives, giving the impression that what she is saying is unimportant, thus reinforcing her insecurities as a communicator and possibly influencing her style to become even more indirect. However, male listeners who do not seem to pay attention might actually be listening for main points while glossing over nonessential details.

Women whose communication includes characteristics that are considered to be "indirect" speech may be viewed by some as weak-willed or ill-equipped for leadership, which could present obstacles to professional advancement. Fortunately, this indirect style of communication is becoming more widely recognized as legitimate in its own right and that not all leadership needs to consistently use direct communication to be effective. For instance, teamwork is often valued by women who emphasize shared leadership, whereas male leaders tend to prefer individualism and hierarchy. Both styles can be highly successful.

FAMILY INTERACTIONS

In family relationships, indirect speech can overlap with indecisive decision making, although the two are not always linked. Some mothers develop a hesitant parenting style, uncertain of their authority over children. They may defer to their husband's authority ("Wait until your father gets home!"). Most moms will agree that they want their children to follow the rules and respect the parents. To reach this goal, parents should use direct speech to be absolutely clear about behavioral expectations and rewards or consequences. However, it is common to hear statements such as the following, often made in a conciliatory tone:

"Please put that candy bar back on the shelf, and I'll get you one later."

(This approach entails bargaining and possible deception if the goal is to divert the child's attention without really buying candy later. A more direct statement is needed: "You've been taught not to touch things that don't belong to you. Put it back.")

"How about cleaning your room before soccer practice?"

(Turning a household rule into a question makes it optional. A statement is emphatic: "Remember to clean your room before soccer practice so you won't be late.")

"I don't think it's a good idea for you to go to an unsupervised party."

(Sharing an opinion is a low-key way to make suggestions without providing guidance or establishing boundaries. Children deserve to know whether they are allowed to do certain things. It is the parent's role to make decisions for underage children: "Unsupervised parties are off limits; too many things can get out of control.")

Household rules need to be spelled out clearly and agreed to by both parents if they reside together or at least enforced by the parent in whose home the child lives or is visiting, if parents are no longer together. Some parents post written rules on the refrigerator or go over a monthly list to discuss how kids are doing in certain areas. The mother sometimes takes parenting cues from the father—even if he is absent, emotionally detached, or overbearing. Often her communication style will attempt to accommodate his, which can work well in certain instances. But at other times one parent is too accommodating, or too competitive, with a confusing and stressful impact on the children.

Indirect speech may be more suitable for teens as they become independent and learn to make personal decisions. But younger children need clear boundaries and rules. Children are quick to note when a parent is unsure and will press the advantage to get what they want. Parents can even be made to feel guilty for being unsure of their position and then give in to the child's request.

"You didn't say no right away, Mom. You know you can trust me."

Of course, a wise parent will point out that a temporary pause means she has given the matter careful consideration, adding weight to her final answer.

Some women take an indirect approach with their spouses, but that can often be more of a personality issue than a communication style. Other women are ultra-clear when they talk to their husbands. As couples learn to amicably live together, they will become more skilled at understanding each other and developing a complementary communication style. They may learn to stop interrupting or arguing with one another and perhaps even begin to complete each other's sentences because their thinking and speaking patterns are in synch.

Long since the Garden of Eden, women are learning to require more information when making important decisions, rather than listen to strangers. Hopefully men will do so, too. Women have learned to speak up and be direct with loved ones, as well as in the business world or in professional endeavors. Moreover, women are holding themselves accountable and expressing sentiments more clearly. Maybe we *have* learned from our mistakes—and those of Adam and Eve. Perhaps a brighter future looms on the horizon for enhanced communication between women and men.

SUGGESTED STRATEGIES

1. If you experience frustration in conversations with the opposite sex, why do you think that is? Spend some time thinking about possible causes of differing communication styles, and take steps to address these in interpersonal communications.
2. As a woman, do you have difficulty speaking up in public? It may help to follow the chain of command (as Eve did not) to get accurate information and make informed decisions.
3. Consider some ways in which you can communicate more directly. Options include using second person instead of an abstract third person and asking for others' input who are involved in the same company projects or sharing your household.

REFERENCES

Bowers, Michael J., and Margaret McCarthy. "'Language Gene' More Active in Young Girls Than Boys." *Science* 22 Dec. 2013: n. pag. Web.

Carter, Sherry Bourg. "High Octane Women." *Psychology Today* 27 Apr. 2011: n. pag. Web.

"Genesis 3." *The Bible*. Bible Gateway. Print.

McCrae, Fiona. "Women Talk Three Times as Much as Men, Says Study." *Daily Mail* 28 Nov. 2006: n. pag. Print.

Mohindra, Vinita and Samina Azhar. "Gender Communication: A Comparative Analysis of Communicational Approaches of Men and Women in Workplaces." *Journal of Humanities and Social Science* 2: 18–27. *iosr journals*. Web. 19 Dec. 2013.

Sholar, Monica Hersh Khetarpal. "Jurors' Perceptions of Gender-Biased Linguistic Differences." *William & Mary Journal of Women and the Law* 10: 90–136. Web. 13 Dec. 2013.

SIX

Whining and Wheedling

Dealing with a toddler's tantrums can grate on anyone's nerves. Just ask a frazzled mom or a busy preschool teacher. Even elementary-age children can become experienced in using whining and wheedling to get their way, quickly noting a caregiver's weaknesses or fatigue. As young children learn to talk, they begin to understand the power of language. Coupled with emotions that often stray beyond civil boundaries, kids' communication can sometimes be direct:

"But I don't wanna take a nap! No-no-no-no!"

"Buy me that candy—PLEASE! I want it—NOW—PLEASE!"

"I won't be tired if I stay up late to watch the movie. I promise."

Although we smile at the memory of expressions like these used by children to get their way, smiles disappear when we hear similar statements from the mouths of adults. A spoiled teen who argues about her homework, a young man who fusses to borrow his parents' car, or a spouse who tries to make deals with the family budget are all annoying, to say the least, as well as risking personal character and family relationships:

"I don't want to do homework before going out with my friends. I should be able to make my own decisions!"

"Please buy me a new car for graduation—PLEASE! All my friends are getting one."

"I'll mow the lawn as soon as this movie is over. I promise."

"We can afford a new Lexus. It won't make a dent in our budget."

Unfortunately, some adults try to bargain for whatever they want instead of directly asking for it with a reasonable explanation. Their approach may include insincere promises, veiled or overt threats, juvenile rebellion, or unfair criticism. Because their efforts have previously been rewarded with success, they continue to use these indirect tactics. For example, an attractive child accustomed to receiving special attention for her looks may continue to use physical appearance as a way to wheedle something from those in authority.

This might include playful or even mildly flirtatious behavior to coerce extra time for a late school assignment or a desired sports team position. Unchecked, actions such as these often progress to seeking workplace favors such as a comfortable job schedule or preferred vacation days. Interpersonal relationships fizzle or operate in a dysfunctional manner if one partner tries to maneuver things his or her way based on personal attributes instead of negotiating important topics toward a win–win resolution.

CHILD WHINERS

Whining is a universal behavior that all of us have witnessed. Usually it is seen in young children who are struggling for attention and self-expression. The *Merriam-Webster Dictionary* defines "whine" as follows:

> to complain in an annoying way
> to make a high, crying sound
> to make a high and unpleasant sound that continues for a long time

Understandably, children whine because of limited communication skills, suggests Beth Halken at babycenter.com:

> Your preschooler relies on adults for almost everything—food, drink, love, you name it. He has to get an adult's attention to obtain the things he needs, and that can be a challenge. Whining is the sound of a child who feels powerless and is pitching his request in higher and higher tones so someone will pay attention to him.

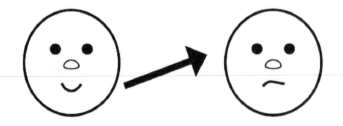

Figure 6.1.   Immature communication in adult conversations: talking "up"

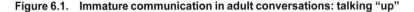

To help children understand why whining is unacceptable, it is important to define the behavior in terms the child can understand and provide examples from television or books with which the child is familiar. Some parents may want to illustrate the behavior, much to children's amusement. Parents should explain that if the child feels he or she is unable to get their attention the regular way, he or she should say so without resorting to whining. This provides a good opportunity to teach children the importance of interrupting a parent's conversation with others only if it is truly important. For example, having to be helped in the bathroom during toilet training is a legitimate reason to seek parental assistance, whereas asking a parent to reach a toy on the top shelf of the closet can probably wait a few minutes. Kids must learn to share parents' attention with others and to seek help appropriately.

Some children—and as we shall see, certain adults—need help in expressing their feelings. Many toddlers whine as a result of fatigue or when they are getting sick. It is important to help a child accurately identify the source of his or her discomfort so she can describe it to a parent or caregiver.

Parents should provide a consistent, calm response that teaches children that whining is unacceptable. This may mean reminding the child to speak in a normal voice or explaining that whining is not acceptable. No matter the parent's mindset or mood, he or she should never give in to the child's whining because that will only teach the child that whining does pay off.

Whining children should be reprimanded and redirected before the behavior becomes unruly. Let's see how these principles apply to adult communication.

ADULT WHINERS

There are different degrees of adult whiners. Some people complain routinely just to vent about the stresses in their lives. This is usually harmless unless they continue to harp endlessly on the same issues over and over, getting on everyone's nerves.

Others get stuck on a particular issue—such as a relationship or job problem—and return to it again and again, wearying longsuffering friends and family members. "Do something about it instead of whining" you want to scream. But folks in this category often seem unable to take decisive action, perhaps doubting their capability or fearing possible consequences. They may need support or reassurance that they are able to analyze relevant facts to make a decision and move forward—even if one option is to make no decision but rather live with the circumstances. That route may at least provide some relief by removing pressure to take action that the person if not ready for.

Some adults whine to close associates as well as virtual strangers. At first thought that may seem odd. But given the growing emotional distance within society today, that is not strange after all.

A column in *The Buffalo News*, "Why Adults Whine and How to Stop Them," suggests two reasons for adult whining, one of which is the desire for connection:

> Sharing your woes with another person makes you feel a little less alone in the world. We want other people to "feel our pain," to share in our ups and downs, and to acknowledge our efforts. This is not a bad thing. When you're feeling down, comforting words from someone who cares can be a soft safe place to land.

When the bank teller asks how your day is going, you may be tempted to tell her about the speeding ticket you just got, the sick child at home, or the thousand errands you have to run that day. Somehow sharing these pressures with someone—anyone—can help to relieve stress and form a temporary bond. We don't feel so alone. We acknowledge shared burdens as part of the human condition. The bank teller in turn may share some of her pressures, and both of you will part ways, each feeling better.

The dark side of these exchanges, however, can descend into narcissism or self-pity, as *The Buffalo News* story notes:

> We (mistakenly) believe that if others truly understood how tough we have it, they'll respect and admire us. Sadly, it doesn't work this way. Telling people how hard things are evokes pity and sympathy at best and boredom and disdain at worst.

We've all had those experiences of standing in line when the person in front of us turns around and begins to complain about the slow service, her aching feet, the weather, or something else that we are helpless to do anything about. Most of us simply smile and nod, not encouraging the conversation, and wonder why the talkative woman is readily opening up to a stranger. Possibly she is lonely or feeling overwhelmed. But after listening to her litany of complaints, criticisms, and concerns, your mood begins to feel dampened, and you really want the line to move quickly so you can get away.

Although whining has been around as long as humankind, some believe it has reached a zenith in contemporary culture, with more adults whining about more issues. From the economy to personal relationships to a host of social concerns, people often verbalize—repeatedly—the things that weigh heaviest on their minds.

Whining in the workplace is becoming increasingly recognized and addressed more aggressively. Here's how one analyst defines it:

> Whining, as defined by experts—the therapists, spouses, co-workers and others who have to listen to it—is chronic complaining, a pattern of negative communication. It brings down the mood of everyone within

earshot. It can hold whiners back at work and keep them stuck in a problem, rather than working to identify a solution. It can be toxic to relationships.

Managers and supervisors now have the authority to institute a no-whining policy in their departments. If they don't have such a policy, they can draft one.

Ron Ashkenas, senior partner of Shaffer Consulting and author of *Simply Effective: How to Cut Through Complexity in Your Organization and Get Things Done*, recommends accountability in discouraging employees from presenting problems without their own attempts at resolution. He also advocates positivity in reminding employees to take a proactive approach when something goes wrong rather than assign blame.

Organizational leaders are expected to set the tone and establish policies for positive communication and interaction. An employee should never whine when asking for a raise, requesting a schedule change, or criticizing a coworker. Whining is counterproductive and a time-waster. Instead, an employee should use a logical, unemotional approach to explain a problem and, if possible, propose a solution that will facilitate a manager's approval. If the employee cannot offer a solution, the problem should be simplified to basic terms that make it convenient to deal with, rather than remain complex and full of emotional ramifications that require digging through layers of verbiage to find core issues. Whining has no meaningful place on the job.

But what can the average person do to deal with someone's constant whining? Showing care and concern is paramount to reassure the person that she is not being rejected. But it is just as important to set healthy boundaries and help her deal responsibly with the troubling issue.

Forty-year-old Karen held up her hand in a "stop" motion when long-time friend Brenda continued to raise the agonizing question of whether to separate from her husband—a conversation they'd had dozens of times—because of her husband's gambling addiction.

> "I realize how important it is to make the right choice, but we've discussed all this before, many times, and it's come down to making the decision to either stay until you feel sure of your feelings or consider possible therapy."

> When Brenda tried to continue the conversation, Karen shook her head with a small smile. "We've covered everything. Just give it a little more thought, make your decision, and then be at peace."

When Brenda realized Karen meant what she said, she stopped complaining and soon did make a decision. Her friendship with Karen remained intact. From that point on she respected her friend's boundaries and learned to be more reserved about whining to other people.

A pair of high school classmates built a friendship based on complementary roles of "whiner" and "listener." Danielle, a lovely blonde-haired, blue-eyed girl used to getting considerable attention at home as the youngest child, complained literally every day that she wasn't pretty enough, her parents didn't really love her, or that her boyfriend was going to cheat on her. Her friend Allison, who wanted to be supportive and help to build Danielle's self-esteem, reassured Danielle constantly that she was the cutest girl in class, that Dakota would never cheat on her, and that her parents were simply looking out for her best interests when they imposed curfews and restrictions. It got to the point that because the two girls exchanged notes at school every day, Allison would write notes the night before, as she did her homework, telling Danielle how pretty she looked and how nice her outfit was—of course insincere and dishonest because they were written before the girls saw each other the following day. She took the shortcut to save time because she knew what was expected, and if she didn't reassure her friend adequately, Danielle would bug her all day by whining.

Unfortunately, Danielle's whining only increased over time. At age seventeen after high school graduation, she got pregnant and married, eventually having three children, three marriages, and three divorces by the time she was thirty. She also became seriously overweight and depressed. The two friends ultimately drifted apart and lost contact, in part because of Danielle's continual whining that Allison could no longer endure.

Sometimes a pair of friends will agree to vent to each other—keeping it brief and focused.

"Hello, Anne? Can I vent about Luke for maybe ten minutes? I don't expect any answers; I just need to get it out of my system."

A "venting partner" can be productive if conversations don't disintegrate into gripe sessions. Ideally, they should be balanced by the friends sharing positives when possible. Otherwise, negativity may breed more negativity; it can become contagious, so that both parties instinctively adopt a bitter attitude when one contacts the other.

If you are continually around someone who wants to whine, don't let it go on endlessly. Just as in responding to preschoolers' whining, we must use proactive strategies to cope with adult whiners. (See Suggested Strategies.)

All of us may feel the need to whine on occasion. We sometimes revert to that former preschool behavior when we get tired or don't feel well. Learning to recognize the signs of whining can help us assert control over an action that has the potential to create problems at work and jeopardize friendships.

WHEEDLING

Merriam-Webster defines "wheedle" as a form of purposeful flattery, to persuade someone to do something or to give you something by saying nice things. To talk someone into doing something may also be described by words such as *charm, coax, finagle, entice, sweet-talk, butter up,* and *work on.* Most of these do not carry pleasant connotations. They imply deceit or delusion that sidesteps honesty and direct dialogue. In fact, the first two definitions of the word *charm* in the *Merriam-Webster Dictionary* suggest supernatural control:

> 1a : the chanting or reciting of a magic spell : incantation
> b: a practice or expression believed to have magic power

Coax, finagle, and *entice* derive from the suggestiveness of luring a victim into a trap.

Thus, to wheedle is not an attractive or admirable practice. It implies cunning meant to trick someone into doing what the speaker wants.

Children, of course, are famous for trying to wheedle things from their parents: more time at a friend's house, a later bedtime, a new toy or treat, or escaping a penalty for misbehavior. Issuing a range of excuses and promises, kids' wheedling can be humorous, although parents should never let on. Generally, wheedling is as annoying as whining, or more so. Smart adults recognize it for what it is, an immature attempt to gain an unwarranted privilege. Wise parents stick to their rules and do not let children manipulate them.

In adults, wheedling can be playful behavior with a purpose:

"If you take me out to dinner, I'll be in a good mood later," a wife promises.

"We can afford a bigger house," an eager husband promises. "I'll get a second job."

"How about making your famous banana cream pie? No one makes it as good as you."

Although there's nothing inherently wrong with the ideas proposed in these statements, the use of wheedling instead of negotiating or debating the pros and cons decreases the likelihood of a meaningful conversation and reasonable outcome. Wheedling is an ages-old method of coercing someone to give us what we want, as depicted in the following scene from Henrik Ibsen's nineteenth-century play, *A Doll's House,* in which wife Nora Helmer tries to convince husband Torvald to give her money as a Christmas gift:

Nora

No, I really can't think of anything—unless, Torvald—

Helmer
Well?

Nora
(playing with his coat buttons, and without raising her eyes to his)
If you really want to give me something, you might—you might—

Helmer
Well, out with it!

Nora
(speaking quickly)
You might give me money, Torvald. Only just as much as you can afford; and then one of these days I will buy something with it.

Helmer
But, Nora—

Nora
Oh, do! dear Torvald; please, please do! Then I will wrap it up in beautiful gilt paper and hang it on the Christmas Tree. Wouldn't that be fun?

Clearly, Nora is trying to wheedle money from her husband. The irony of her plea is that, unknown to Helmer, Nora needs the cash to repay a loan she has illicitly made to support his recovery from a near-fatal illness. The play, published in 1879, raises social awareness of women's limited roles during the time period. By the final scene, Nora and her husband are at last able to have a direct, honest, heart-to-heart conversation about the emptiness of their marriage and Nora's need to discover herself. Former wheedling at the beginning of the play covers a serious legal and marital situation that eventually is revealed, with life-changing consequences. Ibsen highlights the artificial ways in which couples of his era interacted, leaving spouses with just a semblance of contentment and an unhappy longing for self-fulfillment.

Many of us occasionally try to wheedle something, for example, a warning instead of a traffic ticket from a police officer or dodging a committee assignment by saying "you're much better at that sort of thing than I am." Overall, though, it's usually best to be forthright about what we want and why.

In the workplace, wheedling is sometimes used to obtain special consideration:

"I can double our profits by next quarter if you let me have a shot at this project."

"Taking a few days' vacation will let me come back refreshed for next week."

"You're the smartest boss we've ever had, so I know you understand the importance of substantial raises this year."

None of these claims are backed by convincing evidence or measurable results. Repeated requests, empty promises, vague reassurances, and self-gratifying goals are the hallmarks of wheedling behavior. Employees who make requests are more likely to be successful by pitching their proposals in a win–win strategy, acknowledging potential weaknesses and the need for specific resources to reach the goal.

Sometimes sales associates will attempt to wheedle a customer into making a purchase that is not really desired:

"I'll throw in a cover for this appliance if you buy it today."

"We can offer you a lower price if you apply for a store credit card."

"You can easily afford monthly payments on this item."

Smart consumers will carefully balance the proposed advantages against personal shopping goals to determine the merit of the offer. Otherwise, they could be coerced into buying something they don't really want because of the crafty wheedling of a sales associate.

Like other indirect communication practices, wheedling should be avoided. Otherwise, it can put the user in a negative light and result in failure.

SUGGESTED STRATEGIES

1. Deflect chronic whining. Politely remind the whiner by mentioning that the two of you have already discussed the situation. "I realize this is difficult for you, and I wish I could do more to help beyond what we discussed yesterday. Let's see how it goes for the next few days."
2. Set limits. "For your own peace of mind, you don't want to dwell on a negative issue. Let's give it five minutes today, and then focus on something positive."
3. Intercept and redirect. "Still having problems in that area? Did I mention what happened to my friend Elaine? She experienced a similar situation last year and finally found a solution that may interest you."
4. Suggest professional help. "This has been bothering you for several weeks. Do you think it would be helpful to discuss it with a

counselor? I'm sure the experts have more effective advice than I do. Let me help you find a professional therapist."

5. Become an accountability partner. "Timeout, my dear. That's the third time this week you've brought up this topic. Let's talk about something else for a change. I know you don't want to get into a rut and obsess about the situation."

REFERENCES

Ashkenas, Ron. "First Rule of Management: No Whining." *Forbes* 7 Nov. 2012: n. pag. Web.

Bernstein, Elizabeth. "For a Nation of Whiners, Therapists Try Tough Love." *Wall Street Journal* 15 May 2012: n. pag. Web.

"Charm." *Merriam-Webster.com Dictionary*, n.d. Web. 15 Jan. 2014. http://www.merriam-webster.com/dictionary/charm.

Halken, Beth. "Whining: Why it Happens and What to Do about It." babycenter.com, 1 Mar. 2012. Web. 15 Jan. 2014. http://www.babycenter.com/0_whining-why-it-happens-and-what-to-do-about-it_63630.bc.

Ibsen, Henrik. *A Doll's House*. Project Gutenberg, n.d. Web. 15 Jan. 2014. http://www.gutenberg.org/catalog/world/readfile?fk_files=3275005&pageno=1.

"Whine." Merriam-Webster Dictionary, n.d. Web. 15 Jan. 2014. http://www.merriam-webster.com/dictionary/whine.

"Why Adults Whine and How to Stop Them." *The Buffalo News* 1 Dec. 2012, sec. City and Region: n. pag. Print.

SEVEN

Breaking Bad News

Have you ever had the unpleasant task of delivering bad news? Sometimes there is no easy way to say something that will hurt the recipient, such as losing a job or ending a relationship. At other times, the information may be more stressful to the speaker than the listener, as when a student must report failing grades to a parent. Either way, finding the right approach to cushion the blow is a critical component.

Typically, there are two wrong ways to announce bad news: being indirect or being overly direct. Have you ever been confronted by someone who struggled for the right words to tell you something you probably didn't want to hear? The person may have stammered and sputtered to express what needed to be said. Maybe she was overcome by emotion or too timid to say what she knew would be upsetting. Sometimes a person will speak so vaguely that you may have an inkling, but no clear idea, of what is coming. As tension builds, you want to shake the messenger and say, "Out with it!"

Then there's the other type of bad news delivery person who simply states it point blank:

"Your home was broken into, and the thieves took everything."

"Your husband is divorcing you to marry me."

"Your job is being phased out."

Although it's necessary to be made aware of important information, it can be shocking to receive bad news without a buffer.

ELOCUTION VERSUS ELECTROCUTION

Choosing the right words, the best time, and a suitable location to deliver bad news can help to cushion the blow. Just as lightning can strike suddenly without warning, causing irreparable damage, so can unexpected bad news catch someone off-guard and unprepared.

If you must relay disagreeable information, plan carefully for the announcement. A private place is best for news that may be hurtful or disturbing. This could be a private conference room at work or the back porch at home when everyone is out of the way. It is best to avoid building suspense by saying "I have to tell you something bad; can we talk privately?" Rather, use a more neutral invitation: "May I discuss something privately with you? It won't take more than a couple minutes."

Try to choose a time that is not stressful for the recipient. First thing in the morning or just before lunch are not optimum times because people tend to be busy then. Typically, midweek after lunch is a quieter time to share bad news, but not right before a meeting or other commitment.

A middle-aged couple had decided to separate for a time as their marriage began to deteriorate. The preoccupied mom knew she must tell their seventeen-year-old son, but unfortunately chose to do so during the car ride to a photographer for his senior pictures. Although she broke the news as carefully as possible, she will be forever haunted by the hint of sadness in her son's face in all his senior photos. She should have waited to take him aside afterward rather than spoil his mood and his pictures.

In another family, the parents had divorced and the mother was hospitalized for several months with a chronic illness. Her sister, the children's aunt, looked after them during the mother's absence. Soon after, the children were also tested for the contagious illness. A few days later, the aunt, who had been childless up to this time and had little experience in dealing with kids, summoned all four children ranging in age from six to thirteen to the living room and had them sit quietly as she broke more bad news:

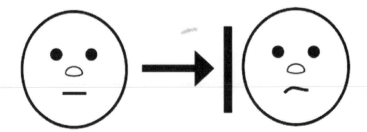

Figure 7.1.   Delivering unwanted information

"One of you has the same condition as your mother. It's not as serious as your mother's case, but it will require taking 21 pills daily. That child must drop out of gym classes and rest after school for a half hour each day."

She stopped, looking around at all four bewildered children. Their father was gone; the mother was hospitalized; what would now happen to the one of them that was also sick? How serious was it? They were too afraid to ask questions, and they did not really understand the situation.

Finally the aunt spoke. "It's you, Leah," she said, nodding at the oldest with a slight smile. The thirteen-year-old felt as though she had received a death sentence.

"Me?" she stuttered.

"Yes, but you will be fine if you take your pills and do what you're supposed to."

Although the aunt meant well in being direct with the children about the illness, her approach actually frightened them. It took several days before they realized that Leah would not be taken from the family as their mother had been. The aunt's revelation could have been handled in a more low-key way to avoid traumatizing the kids. But as a nurse, that was the aunt's only experience in how to deliver bad news—swiftly and directly.

Fortunately, the mother and daughter recovered, and the aunt did a good job of parenting the children for the next eight months. Still, her way of announcing bad news continued to be almost extreme, although the children began to take her warnings less seriously.

When sharing bad news, it is important to consider the listener's age and education or socioeconomic background. Some people are better equipped to receive bad tidings, whereas others quickly get scared and even panic without adequate cushioning. Without mincing words, it is usually a good idea to speak directly but not in a dire manner, especially with those who are potentially fragile, including children, the elderly, and very ill people. If possible, temper the bad news with a neutral or positive statement to make the revelation more bearable. For example, if someone must be told of a health crisis, it is helpful to offer support and encouragement. Also, when possible, place the bad news part of a statement in a subordinate clause rather than a main clause:

Main clause: "You have a serious diagnosis."
Subordinate clause: "Although you have a serious diagnosis, . . ."

Add the positive part of the statement in a main clause that follows the subordinate clause: "Although it is a serious diagnosis, you have a great medical team."

ON THE JOB

Most of us are accustomed to receiving bad news occasionally. In fact, in these uncertain times, it's not unusual to get bad news about others or loved ones on a fairly routine basis. Falling stocks, lost jobs, and home foreclosures are widespread. Even a solid employment record is no guarantee against a disappointing turn of events. Robert J. Bies of Georgetown University explains in his article "The Delivery of Bad News in Organizations" that bad news may be defined as "information that results in a perceived loss by the receiver, and it creates cognitive, emotional, or behavioral deficits in the receiver after receiving the news." He emphasizes that receiving bad news can become, for many, an "almost daily phenomenon" in the workplace. Bad news on the job is certainly difficult to handle, especially while maintaining a professional demeanor.

Unfortunately, some employers wait to drop the "F" (fired) bomb until Friday at 5 p.m. to avoid any emotional fallout that may follow. An employee who has no advance warming of losing her job may be shocked to be told at the end of the week that she need not return. This is a case of being too blunt without due process of providing the employee with the opportunity of improving job performance to keep the position or looking for another job before the current one ends.

On the other end of the spectrum, some supervisors only hint at dissatisfaction with an employee's job performance. They assume the employee will figure it out through occasional criticisms leveled his or her way and make appropriate changes. When that doesn't happen, as a result of the supervisors' indirect communication style, employees are stumped to learn their job is on the line when appraisal time rolls around. Suddenly, they are accused of unsuitable work habits and failing to respond to supervisors' recommendations, when the "recommendations" were vague verbal suggestions to "try a little harder" or "work a little faster." The typical employee might interpret such comments as a supervisor's temporary bad mood or referring to just that day, not overall performance. That is why it is important for supervisors to keep clear written records for performance appraisals and go over them in detail with each employee at least once a year. Employees should then have the opportunity to ask questions or request clarification, along with the opportunity to improve and thus keep their jobs.

Job performance evaluations should be written descriptively to help supervisors and employees identify specific work-related behaviors for review. These assessment criteria may become the basis for good news or bad news, but in either case, they need to be clearly understood by both supervisor and employee. Here are a few examples:

Table 7.1.

Vague:	Specific:
Works well with others	Cooperative and productive team player
Good attendance	Misses one day or less per month for acceptable reasons
Positive attitude	Gets along well with employees and supervisors
Accepts criticism	Responds constructively to criticism with efforts to improve

Accompanied by a numerical scoring range, such as 1 through 10 (with 1 being poor and 10 being excellent), criteria such as these can help employees and supervisors track job performance in tandem, providing well-defined areas of concern or success. When a supervisor indicates a category is average or needs work, specific examples for improvement should be given to encourage the employee to try harder.

Sometimes an employee is reprimanded for workplace behavior. This would be construed as bad news, presumably deserved. Even so, employee morale can be maintained by indicating the route by which a weakness can be overcome or a problem avoided in the future. This approach helps to buffer the negative impact of bad news and provide an opportunity for improvement that can lead to good news at the next performance appraisal.

Worksite counselors and organizational psychologists often assist employees in navigating bad news developments, from a change in job duties to decreased pay. Of course, professional counselors and therapists in the public sector can likewise help. Clear communication helps to alleviate unpleasant surprises and frustrating disappointments, as long as the message is not cold or calloused, and includes some cushioning to soften the negative impact.

In fact, failure—reported as bad news—often becomes the impetus for change, leading eventually to improvement and success.

How terrible it must feel to fail in front of millions. Yet, sports celebrities use their disappointing plays to work even harder and become the athletic superstars they are destined to be.

How many lost fortunes, organizational scandals, and incalculable losses have been reported as bad news? Although some people have received devastating circumstances by sinking into despair or committing suicide, others have survived and grown stronger to eventually succeed in new endeavors. Bad news should not be viewed as falling into an abyss, but rather as the beginning of building a bridge to cross the abyss.

PERSONAL RELATIONSHIPS

On the home front, shifting cultural values have led to more unstable and short-term relationships, with fewer marriages that often end more quickly than in generations past. Although some hail this trend as a hallmark of greater personal freedom, it should be acknowledged that a string of short, failed relationships generally leave people dissatisfied or unhappy—not to mention the potential negative effects on children living in a revolving-door environment.

Do you know anyone who can nonchalantly accept a statement like "I don't love you anymore"? Of course, if the hearer feels the same way, there may be a sense of relief. Otherwise, it is painful to hear this and feel helpless to change the speaker's feelings.

How can bad news of this type be candidly delivered without seeming calloused?

Hurtful announcements should not come out of nowhere. After all, destructive words have the power to kill a relationship or douse someone's spirit. Ideally, one or both persons will sense a persistent problem and make efforts to address it before the issue becomes irreconcilable. Most of us fall in and out of love with a mate fairly regularly. One day he looks perfect, and the next you question your sanity for marrying him. But when a situation begins to fester, leading to depression and anger, dealing with it responsibly instead of sweeping it under the carpet can head off potential disaster.

"We seem unable to get past this roadblock. Let's make an appointment with a therapist."

"I just feel like our marriage isn't working anymore. Can we work on it?"

An insecure person might take statements such as these to be the kiss of death to a relationship. Actually, these are the words that may save a troubled marriage. For example, medical practitioners are trained to speak directly with patients about conditions that are serious, or even terminal. It's only fair for sick people to know exactly what is wrong, as well as receive a professional opinion on the outlook, to help them prepare for the future. Couples in endangered relationships should give each other the same consideration—with care and compassion.

Because emotions can get wildly out of control, it is important to plan what you want to say, and how best to say it, before speaking. Of course, it is wise to avoid sweeping generalizations:

"You make me sick! I can't stand you! Your spending is out of control!"

Instead, focus on one specific problem that can be reasonably addressed:

"We need to discuss our finances. When is a good time to do that?"

"The kids are getting to bed too late. Let's decide how to get them back on schedule."

Statements like these are nonthreatening and yet specific, suggesting a productive way of dealing with problems. If a couple is unable to be civil with each other or cannot identify a target problem, they may need the assistance of a professional counselor. Learning effective communication skills can provide the tools needed to deal with a wider range of issues that may be too complicated or sensitive for a couple to handle on their own.

Bad news is usually a source of discomfort for the messenger as well as the recipient. Those reporting unhappy information may be the bearer of announcements about employee performance reviews, customer dissatisfaction, or company downsizing. Consequently, they face the potential for retaliation, earning others' bias and distrust. You've probably heard the saying, "Don't shoot the messenger," which suggests that recipients of bad news have been known to lash out at the hapless agent. If we can't attack the source of the problem, we'll settle for the delivery guy. Although we like to think of ourselves as civilized, maybe you can recall a time when someone gave you unpleasant information and you reacted in a rude manner.

Someone who tells a friend about her husband's infidelity may be treated coldly by the wife, and some friendships are even severed. This is not because the wife distrusts the friend who reveals the disturbing news, but because the news is so hurtful the wife pushes away anyone connected to it. Later, those damaged friendships may be repaired, though some never are.

The same rejecting response sometimes occurs when neighbors report a child's bad behavior to the parent. Not wanting others to discredit her child, a mother often chooses to believe her child's untruth about his actions rather than accept the neighbor or teacher's account. Parental reluctance stems from protectiveness, disbelief, or negligence. Many neighborhood feuds and classroom disputes at parent–teacher conferences have ensued when a parent refused to accept bad news about a child. Of course, if the charge is true, a parent who refuses to consider the accusation unwittingly supports the child's ongoing misbehavior. Too many parents interpret criticism against a child as leveled at them, and thus go on the defensive to protect their good name as much as the child's reputation. Although it's important to believe in a child and stand up for her when warranted, it is also vital for parents to let children be held accountable for their actions.

INDIRECT BAD NEWS

Some people cannot bring themselves to directly report bad news to the appropriate person, whether a supervisor or close friend. They resort to slandering the alleged offender to share their outrage indirectly with others. Hints, gossip, and innuendo "leak" bad news that someone does not want to address directly.

Those who find conflict unbearable sometimes use sarcasm to make a point:

"Don't worry about making breakfast tomorrow, since you enjoy sleeping in so much."

Instead of asking a spouse to get up and make breakfast or help with getting the kids off to school, the stressed spouse will avoid confrontation and snipe at the other person instead. This only increases tensions and makes it harder to deal with the core issues.

Others simply refuse to bring up any negative topics. They don't stand up for themselves or address a perceived slight, leaving the offender in the dark. Then, as the victim grows increasingly offended, she explodes one day, bringing up every bad thing the person did (in her opinion because these things were never discussed or explained) in an all-out attack. Usually this response causes a breach in the relationship that often is temporary but may be permanent. I have known two daughters who had a dispute with their father while in their teens and refused to talk to him for the next forty years. It's far better to deal with each perceived affront as it occurs, although a brief cooling-down period may be advisable first, rather than letting many such occurrences build up and lead to an explosion of conflict at some point, possibly causing irreparable damage.

Bad news is no fun for anyone. But because it is part of life, we should learn to deal with it as sensibly as possible. Don't be taken by surprise. The next time you have to deliver—or receive—bad news, exercise self-control in your response to achieve a suitable outcome.

Telling someone what they don't want to hear is often unpleasant for both messenger and listener. But not all negative messages have to be devastating. A thoughtful messenger can learn to cushion the blow.

SUGGESTED STRATEGIES

When delivering bad news, consider the following approaches, many of which are widely used in the business world and in counseling situations. They may help the hearer to better receive a negative message.

1. Be sensitive to the recipient. Based on available information, try to anticipate how the hearer will accept the message. Determine if possible whether she is likely to be angry, frustrated, sad, and so on. Shape your message accordingly. If you know, for example, that the person—your friend—has been having ongoing relationship problems with her boyfriend, you will want to be aware of the fact that she may be emotional on the subject. Stick to the facts, and reveal only as much as is needed. There is a story floating around about a tired and discouraged-looking man who gets on the bus with two children. The kids romp up and down the aisle, annoying several passengers as they whisk past and giggle loudly. An older woman who had raised her family with firm discipline took a moment as the bus reached her stop to urge the father to better control his children. The man looked up sadly as she finished speaking and said, "I'm sorry, ma'am. I've just come from the hospital where my wife died and was distracted. I'll keep a better eye on them." Had the woman read the "clues" in the father's face or asked if everything was all right, she could have spared him discomfort and herself some embarrassment.

2. Choose the best time and place. Clearly, delivering bad news in the grocery checkout line is not prudent. Doing so while riding in a car with someone may not be wise because the person is "trapped" with you (and any other passengers) until you reach the destination. It may be difficult for the recipient to share an honest response.

   Instead, choose a private place at a time that does not compete with other activities. Telling a neighbor that her daughter just hit a baseball through a window and broke it as the neighbor is leaving for work will probably add to her stress load for the day. After dinner or during another low-key time in the person's schedule will help to reduce tension. A face-to-face meeting is preferable, with a phone call a secondary option. Texting or e-mail is less direct, and some people take such messages less seriously.

3. Decide which aspects of the message need to be shared. If minor details can wait, it might be best to focus only on the main point.

For example, if the neighbor's dog keeps wandering into your yard and digging up the flower beds, you don't necessarily have to say how much the flowers cost (unless you are seeking compensation) or when they were planted. Simply state the frequency of the dog's trespassing and the flowers being damaged. Details can be added as needed. Keep the message simple to avoid getting bogged down in small points that may be irrelevant.

4. Be respectful. If you are sharing a problem that involves you (as opposed to being just the messenger of others' concerns), use integrity. Avoid trigger words that label, criticize, or belittle the other person. Display patience and understanding. In classical times, and even today in sporting competitions, opponents typically acknowledge each other with a bow, nod, or handshake. This shows that both sides recognize the opponent's merit and equality. Imagine neighborhoods, homes, and workplaces where name-calling, yelling, and insults were absent. If we handled everyday conflicts respectfully, the world would be much saner—and safer.

5. Balance negatives with positives. In some cases this is impossible, for example, when someone dies. Even then, we sometimes hear comments like, "At least he won't be suffering anymore" or "He died doing what he loves" (as in a sporting accident), although some grief experts question the validity of such statements. Sometimes all we can do is offer comfort and consolation.

   However, in other cases, it may be possible to cushion the blow with a few hopeful ideas. This doesn't mean we should minimize the truth, but rather help the hearer to see the big picture. For example, if a mother who is working full-time has her hours cut, she might be encouraged to reconfigure her budget to reduce costs while enjoying more time at home with her children, even if it just until she finds a second job. (Most likely only a close friend or relative could say this, and only at the right time.) Learning of a child's misbehavior at a minimal level lets a parent deal with it before the problem gets out of hand. For example, instead of saying, "I caught your son in a lie," it is probably better to say that "Johnny's facts seem unclear; can we discuss the situation?"

6. Be a good listener. Give the recipient of the bad news the opportunity to respond. Erika Andersen, *Forbes* contributor, discusses this step that should be followed by business leaders. "Don't try to talk people out of being upset. Once you've let a big cat out of a big bag, you need to let people say what they think and feel about it."

   Think how it would feel to be punched in the face and then forced to be silent. Certain types of bad news significantly impact the brain's pain center. Without an outlet for releasing that pain, hearers will only feel worse. Although you may not normally be a close confidante of the person, the recipient might want to express a gut-level response before venting in expansive ways with loved ones and friends.

7. Offer guidance. Depending on circumstances, this might not be possible. But if you can suggest a possible solution or at least a resource to consult, that might ease the burden of managing a new problem or loss. One example is when a supervisor privately confronts an employee about drinking on the job. The positive side of the conversation would be to suggest help for the employee, some of which may be company-paid, such as counseling, whereas other resources are free, such as AA. Offering assistance shows compassion and alleviates some of the strain of receiving bad news.

REFERENCES

Andersen, Erika. "How Great Leaders Deliver Bad News." *Forbes* 6 Mar. 2013: n. pag. Web.

Bies, Robert J. "The Delivery of Bad News in Organizations." *Journal of Management*: n. pag. *Journal of Management*. Web. 19 Jan. 2014.

EIGHT

Signs and Signals

An anxious twenty-two-year-old texted her sister at home: "Is the Camry still there?"

The sister texted back, "Yep" followed by a smiley face as a token of reassurance.

The first texter's concern stemmed from an argument she and her boyfriend had just had. He had demanded the return of the Camry loaned her until she graduated with a nursing degree and could buy her own car. Mark had directed his now "ex-girlfriend" to leave the 2004 Camry in her sister's driveway for his later retrieval. Tonia did so. Now, hours later, she was trying to find out if Mark had truly finalized their breakup by taking back the car.

For this couple, the Camry became a tangible symbol of their relationship. Once Mark actually reclaimed the car, both would consider the relationship finished. The next day, Tonia texted her sister to ask about the car, but Mark had not come for it. By the third day, Mark texted Tonia to ask if she had parked the vehicle as directed. Of course, his text message to Tonia was a pretense for reestablishing communication, and within an hour, the couple had made up. Later that day, Mark dropped off Tonia at her sister's to retrieve the car. Reclaiming the Camry signified the reinstatement of their relationship.

For some, negotiating in material goods is easier than navigating emotions. For instance, the engagement ring is a universal symbol of commitment leading to marriage. But for many couples, not just any ring will do. Some women expect, or even demand, a certain quality or price tag: it must be at least a full carat or cost at least $5,000. Similarly, the man may feel pressure to provide a specific standard of ring for his fiancée. The ring comes to represent a variety of things for those buying and wearing it:

- Socioeconomic status of the groom, bride, or both
- Significance of the relationship
- Valuation of the bride by the groom
- Bride's success in attracting a financially secure mate

Jewelry speaks a language of its own, usually of a romantic or commemorative nature, to celebrate engagements, weddings, births, and anniversaries. Ironically, there are marriages where a cheating husband, when caught, buys his wife an expensive diamond bracelet as a symbolic apology. When the wife accepts this token gesture, she may be tacitly expressing forgiveness of the breach or even passively implying she will tolerate infidelity as long as she receives "hush money" in the form of costly gifts.

After couples wed, establish a home, and raise a family, their material possessions often become the gauge of not only their financial status, but also the measure of their mutual affection.

"Oh, he is crazy about her! Look at that beautiful home he built."

"He makes sure she drives only late-model cars."

"If he really loved her, he would support her with a decent standard of living."

"She left her husband for a man who earns more money."

Eventually, as some marriages come to an end, the devaluation of the family unit and the inflation of the sense of self lead to conflict over who gets to keep what in the division of marital assets. In place of loving words, embraces, and vows spoken before witnesses to proclaim a lifelong commitment, the relationship disintegrates to desperate bargaining between divorce attorneys behind closed doors to give each "party" (formerly, spouse) the once-shared possessions that now mean more than the person that each professed to love. Division of possessions represents the fragmentation of the union.

Even the children can be treated like chattel, as self-absorbed parents fight over visitation rights, custody disputes, and child support. Although offspring are often initially viewed as a token of love between parents, too often they sadly become the leftover afterthoughts of a hurting couple so deeply focused on their individual needs that they are unable to thoughtfully consider the best interests of the children.

When conflicts become heated, reason goes out the window. Instead of problem-solving in a rational way, such as using direct communication to reasonably discuss relevant issues, we affix meaning to symbolic objects that cannot argue or take sides. They can simply be transferred in ownership, like chess pieces on a game board, to reflect the players' moves.

COMMUNICATING WITH SIGNS

Perhaps more than we realize, we interact daily with others through a variety of signs and signals, all of which carry representative meaning. The success of this form of communication depends on the shared understanding of a sign's meaning. Print, Web, and radio or TV advertisements strive to make their point in a brief glimpse; thus, a symbolic message must be able to reach—and influence—the largest possible number of readers, listeners, or viewers. When this happens, the ad is successful. But when it doesn't, the message fails.

Semiotics is a theory of language that studies the ability of signs and symbols to artificially and naturally represent meaning between a message's sender and recipient. According to philosopher and semiotics researcher Umberto Eco, the sign's representative meaning may be real or abstract:

> A sign is everything which can be taken as significantly substituting for something else. This something else does not necessarily have to exist or to actually be somewhere at the moment in which a sign stands for it (7).

Thus, a sign theoretically could represent a real or imagined idea. Because each of us is designed uniquely, it can be challenging to use symbolic words or gestures with those who may not grasp their intent. Meanings may be misunderstood, adding to confusion or conflict.

How widespread is the use of signs? According to Eco, "There is a sign every time a human group decides to use and to recognize some-

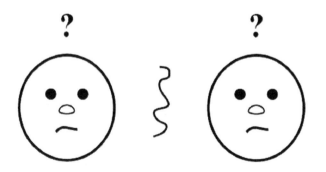

Figure 8.1. Interpretative symbolism

thing as the vehicle of something else" (17). Because we do not communicate literally one hundred percent of the time, it is probably safe to say that most of us use communicative symbolism on a regular basis, possibly without realizing it. The potential for misunderstanding is considerable, especially across cultures. This explains some of the constant tensions between individuals or groups who fail to comprehend certain symbols or signs.

Indeed, objects play a strategic role in various interactions and relationships. From the aforementioned jewelry to transferred ownership of objects, signs replace spoken language in meaningful and not-so-meaningful ways. Have you ever received a gift that was definitely not what you wanted? Evidently the giver hoped to express appreciation but failed to understand that the gift did not have the same meaning for you as it did for her. Family heirlooms, such as a World War II military uniform or a hundred-year-old Singer sewing machine, might be prized by one family member but disdained by another. Wearing a grandmother's retro wedding dress will appeal to some young ladies, but not all. An object's symbolic value is variable rather than fixed.

Ironically, the absence of signs reveals much about a person's character or a relationship. More broadly, signs and signals are the mechanisms of communication that allow people to interact in representative ways. Robert M. Krauss explains this purpose:

> Communication systems use two kinds of signals: signs and symbols. Signs are signals that are causally related to the message they convey. We say that blushing means someone is embarrassed because we know that embarrassment is a cause of blushing. Symbols, on the other hand, are products of social conventions.

When a friend's face turns red and his brows become furrowed, you assume he is angry. A woman who turns away with slumped shoulders might appear defeated or sad. Without knowing more about the situation, however, it can be difficult to know for sure how to interpret a person's behavior. Shared context facilitates sign-oriented communication. Without context, speakers and listeners must take into consideration the possible backdrop necessary to understand the intended message. Winking may come across as flirtatious to some or encouraging to others. A hug might be construed as supportive or intrusive, depending on context.

We cannot always assume that signs or signals will be interpreted the way we want them to be. When in doubt it is best to ask rather than assume. In their book *Social Semiotics*, Robert Hodge and Gunther Kress emphasize the importance of shared understanding for interpreting symbolic language:

> Each producer of a message relies on its recipients for it to function as intended. This requires these recipients to have knowledge of a set of

messages on another level, messages that provide specific information about how to read the message. (4)

In short, unless sender and receiver perceive the symbolic message in a similar manner, its meaning will be lost. As Hodge and Kress explain, "The message has directionality—it has a source and a goal, a social context and a purpose" (5). But there are no simple explanations for personal signs and symbols.

Human nature tells us that we believe what we want to believe. History, context, and emotions play a role in the translation of signs when words (direct communication) are absent or few. When an attractive single man in his early thirties gave a single red rose to the single ladies on his bowling team on Valentine's Day, some found the gesture sweet, whereas two women interpreted it as possible romantic interest. It turned out the man had been prompted by a friend to do a "good deed" for the single ladies as an act of encouragement, nothing more.

Similar instances can be found in literature. "The Necklace," a short story published in 1884 by French author Guy de Maupassant, is based on the incorrect assumption of a young woman who borrows a friend's necklace to wear to a party, loses it, and replaces it—unknown to her friend—at a price that requires ten years of hard work to repay. Ironically, she encounters the friend ten years later and learns the original necklace was a cheap imitation. If only Madame Loisel had inquired about the jewelry's true value before assuming otherwise! The necklace objectifies Madame Loisel's impression of her friend's wealth, resulting in a huge burden of debt and wasted youth spent working to repay the symbolic object's false worth.

How often do we similarly misinterpret the value of objects in our lives, and the lives of those around us, leading to miscommunication? When a ten-year-old child is given a cell phone for personal use, how will her teachers and classmates interpret the object? Is the phone meant to be used as a security device only in case of emergencies, or rather to become a social construct as the girl develops friendships through texting and phone conversations? Will others view her parents as protective? Or will they perceive the child to be spoiled and perhaps inadequately supervised?

ATTITUDES OBJECTIFIED

We live in a culture that uses signs to represent a wide spectrum of meanings—meanings that continue to expand, change, and disappear over time:

From the moment children are born, perhaps from a time before then, they are subject to the effects of semiosis and culture. The new-born

> [sic] enter at once into a semiotic relationship with other humans
> around them and, in a process which ceases only at death, they con-
> struct a world of meaning, and are constructed by an already-semioti-
> cized world. The process is constantly interactive and dynamic . . .
> (Hodge and Kress 240)

From gestures to facial expressions and physical objects to actions, we
learn from an early age how to represent meaning in ways that will
influence others. Toddlers soon understand the meaning of "no" as a
word when supported by an action, like being removed from a spot near
the stove. Few parents tell their teens, "I don't care what you do; get into
any trouble you want." School-age children learn whether parents are
interested in their academic progress by the attention spent on supervis-
ing homework or involvement in school activities. Teens are quick to
read preoccupation with jobs or social activities as a signal that inatten-
tive parents are likelier to overlook the kids' problem behaviors. Actions
can be just as symbolic, or more so, as words.

As we come of age and begin to understand the value of money, we
realize that it is a medium for obtaining things we desire. In fact, material
goods come to represent much of who we are or want to be. Money used
to purchase tangible objects is often the basis for evaluating someone's
value or performance. We have already discussed the symbolism of engagement rings and briefly touched on the implications of expensive possessions. A pricy house or luxury car may be purchased for showy qualities as much as comfort. Likewise, those with low-status possessions
such as a beater car or a modest home may be rated as inferior by those in
higher social standing. Yet, those with cheaper material goods may actually be saving more money and investing in the future more than their
neighbors who buy expensive things.

Interestingly, the absence of clear verbal cues sends its own subliminal
message. A factory that is rife with safety violations creates dangerous
working conditions for employees. What does that suggest about management's attitude? Schools with broken windows, poorly paid teachers,
and out-of-date textbooks send a powerful message about the low value
placed on education. Although professional sports play an important role
in the entertainment industry and as a legitimate recreational outlet, a
comparison of salaries and work conditions of educated teachers and
trained athletes raises provocative questions about which group is valued
more by society.

Kids that come to school poorly dressed or hungry raise red flags
about their home life, without speaking a word. At the very least, we
suspect the family must be struggling. At worst, the children may be
suffering neglect. The same interpretations apply to the senile elderly and
the mentally challenged who are unable to communicate clearly. We
learn to read the surrounding circumstances and render a judgment.

Signs and signals are everywhere, used by the entertainment industry in films and music, advertising and marketing gurus in ads of various kinds, medical professionals in reading disease symptoms, and fashion experts whose designs emulate or influence culture. If a financial analyst misreads stock market cues and provides the wrong advice, investors could lose significant holdings. Doctors who mistakenly interpret a patient's symptoms may prescribe the wrong treatment. Impressionable preteens or teenagers may mistakenly interpret a pop song's lyrics as supportive of drug use, violence, or suicide when the song is sarcastically criticizing these actions.

In the physical communication realm, signs and signals flourish. Many are age-old traditions, such as a goodnight kiss or a wave of the hand, whereas others provide discreet ways of sharing delicate information, such as physical touch or a loving smile. Toddlers learn that a nighttime story is the prelude to bedtime. Food rituals often play a role, from Saturday morning breakfast in bed to a Sunday afternoon drive to the ice cream stand. These practices build and sustain relationships without anyone saying as much.

Dr. Gary Chapman's book, *The Five Love Languages*, discusses five important types of interaction that convey a sense of love. An online *Personality Cafe* article explains these communication styles and points out that acts of service will substitute actions for words:

> People who speak this love language seek to please their partners by serving them; to express their love for them by doing things for them. Actions such as cooking a meal, setting a table, washing the dishes, sorting the bills, walking the dog or dealing with landlords are all acts of service. They require thought, planning, time, effort and energy. If done with a positive spirit, they are indeed expressions of love.

Without a word, a wife or husband can clearly demonstrate affection by performing actions that benefit the other spouse. Although acts of service may seem like an indirect form of communication, they are actually strong, vibrant expressions of caring. There can be little doubt on the recipient's part of the giver's meaning.

Objects, gifts, attitudes, and actions convey meaning apart from language. Just as we should work at being effective listeners, we should also strive to correctly understand others' behavior that impacts us.

SYMBOLIC GESTURES

Meta-communication, or body language, involves a variety of facial expressions, bodily movements, and stance that convey meaning, purposefully or unconsciously. Here are some universal examples:

- Smile or frown

- Wink
- Shrug
- Folded arms
- Hand gestures
- Shaking head up and down or side to side
- Volume and clarity of speech

There are many more. Whether a person faces you or turns away while conversing, if she slumps or stands erect, and other aspects of physical interaction help to translate a person's actual thoughts or feelings.

In-depth emotions are sometimes expressed through extended behavior. In a previous chapter we discussed the silent treatment. Sometimes a person who is angry will deliberately come home late to upset a spouse. A person may refuse to handle her usual household chores; for example, a wife who becomes irate over her husband's leaving dirty clothes on the floor might stop picking up the clothes and let the laundry go unwashed—to send a symbolic message. This can occur in the workplace as well, with a disgruntled employee adopting a passive-aggressive attitude toward her workload as a form of noncompliance. The phenomenon of "blue flu," when uniformed officers (often police) call in sick to protest job policies, shares this behavior throughout an entire department or organization to make a "statement" of solidarity.

In the professional realms, signals play a valuable role in helping team members or coworkers to communicate across a large area or over a noisy background. Restaurant servers, sports team members, and military personnel use a specific set of signals, a nonverbal communication code, to relay important information. In classrooms, nonverbal signals can stimulate metacognitive strategies for intellectual engagement and problem-solving activities. One example is a clicker used to let students electronically signal a response to a question without being individually identified. Instructors believe that clickers promote more student interaction when students can anonymously participate, especially those that are unsure or self-conscious. Thus, education may be enhanced through nonverbal interaction.

Recent scientific study of micro-expressions, which are uncontrolled facial movements lasting a fraction of a second to subconsciously convey one of the principal emotions (anger, love, fear, sadness), also contribute to "reading" a person's inner feelings, despite the effort to present a "poker" face. Here is a definition from the American Psychological Association:

> When single emotions occur and there is no reason for them to be modified or concealed, expressions typically last between 0.5 to 4 seconds. (Matsumoto and Hwang)

We call these macro-expressions; they occur whenever we are alone or with family and close friends. Macro-expressions are relatively easy to see if one knows what to look for. Micro-expressions, however, are expressions that flash on and off the face in a fraction of a second, sometimes as fast as one-thirtieth of a second. They are so fast that if you blink you would miss them.

Micro-expressions are likely signs of concealed emotions. (They may also be signs of rapidly processed but unconcealed emotional states.) They occur so fast that most people cannot see or recognize them in real time.

Symbolic gestures, that is, gestures or actions that knowingly or unknowingly hold meaning for the giver or receiver, are frequently used in place of verbal communication.

Sometimes a poster or print sign says it all. In Appalachia, an aging, independent man who lived alone in a rural area was warned by local law enforcement about the rowdy drug users who bought a nearby piece of land. The rugged mountaineer didn't respond directly to the officer's warning, but soon a 12"x10" wooden sign was posted on his front porch railing depicting a mountaineer holding a shotgun with the words "We don't call 9-1-1." The implication was that the man would personally handle any threats before calling for help.

Although sentimental signs and signals can be heart-warming and are often preferred in personal relationships over flat-line direct communication, it is important that nonverbal messages be designed in ways that will be clear to recipients. In the professions, clear communication is as vital for success as it is for the survival of interpersonal relationships.

Language signals play an important role in communication. Some are so widespread that most of us automatically understand their meaning. Others are new or personalized and require thought or interpretation. It is critical to ensure that the receiver of a message based on signs, signals, or symbols will grasp its meaning.

We often find it difficult to "read" people when unconventional communication styles are used. By learning to better understand the nuances of unspoken communication, along with implied meanings of gestures or objects, we have a better chance of perceiving their meaning and can ourselves transmit more effective messages in a style that receivers can appreciate.

In general, it is best to use signs sparingly unless they are intended to serve a specific purpose. Objects, codes, and documents that are meant to be symbolic may end up falling short of their purpose and cause confusion.

SUGGESTED STRATEGIES

1. Consider what the recipient already knows about the topic. Will background information or context be needed? For example, sending an unrequested photo of yourself to a newfound acquaintance on social media can be interpreted in various ways. Will it be understood as a romantic outreach or as a casual invitation to get better acquainted?

2. Decide if the message could be misunderstood. Factors such as gender, age, education, and socioeconomic background should come into play. If you send a coworker who is about to retire a cartoon about an elderly person, the reader may think the cartoon is intended as a comment about her age.

3. Could direct communication better serve the purpose? A cryptic message or a symbolic object can be meaningful if understood, or confusing if not. It's important to be on comfortable terms with someone before using signs and signals they may not understand. For example, Ron had been discussing spiritual views with coworker Tara and wanted to invite her to church. On Monday morning he left his weekly church bulletin on her desk to pique her interest. However, when Tara saw the bulletin, she thought Ron was making a judgmental accusation about her differing religious background and felt insulted. When she became less friendly around Ron, he didn't understand, and the budding friendship fizzled.

4. Make sure the symbolism is clear. Unless you are confident the receiver of your signal clearly "gets" its intended message, it's probably helpful to follow up and offer explanation if needed: "Did the article I forwarded make sense?"

5. How should the message be conveyed? Choose a suitable format. It is probably best not to send a message of uncommon acronyms via text, which, as a result of brevity, may add to potential confusion. Playful expressions or mysterious phrasing should be reserved for face-to-face interactions, where meta-communication (i.e., body language) can help a listener to decipher the meaning. E-mail or written messages (such as a greeting card or letter) provide more area space for explanations. Texting or social media posts work well with messages that don't require intricate interpretation. Social networking should not be laced with special signs or hidden meanings, unless, of course, the goal is to deliberately exclude others.

REFERENCES

Eco, Umberto. *A Theory of Semiotics*. Bloomington: Indiana UP, 1979. Print.

Hodge, Robert and Gunther Kress. *Social Semiotics*. Ithaca: Cornell UP, 1988. Print.

Krauss, Robert M. "The Psychology of Verbal Communication." N. Smelser, and P. Baltes, eds. *The International Encyclopedia of the Social and Behavioral Sciences*. Columbia University. 1 Jan. 2002. Web. 8 Feb. 2014. http://www.columbia.edu/~rmk7/PDF/IESBS.pdf.

Matsumoto, David and Hyi Sung Hwang. "Reading Facial Expressions of Emotion." American Psychological Association, 1 May 2011. Web. 11 Feb. 2014. http://www.apa.org/science/about/psa/2011/05/facial-expressions.aspx.

"The 5 Love Languages Explained." Personality Cafe, 21 Aug. 2012. Web. 11 Feb. 2014. http://personalitycafe.com/articles/112444-five-love-languages-explained.html.

NINE

Say Less and Mean More

How many books have ever been published *in all of modern history?* According to Google's advanced algorithms, the answer is nearly 130 million books, or 129,864,880, to be exact. (Google)

That's quite a few books in print. According to Amazon's Text Stats feature, the average book length is 64,000 words, which totals to a mind-boggling number of words in publication today. Some experts consider this figure to be low, and it doesn't include audio recordings, video recordings, and other media using words as their communication medium, such as articles, pamphlets, newsletters, and so on.

Yet, how many people have read even 10 percent of all published books? Assuming most people have not, that's a lot of unused verbiage. If we were able to read a significant portion of the books in print, we would gain a great deal of knowledge, along with exposure to countless ideas, many of which might be unvalued by a majority as their usefulness and applicability to each person's life would vary. So, even though billions of printed words are circulating today, it's safe to say that most are not read by the majority of the population.

Now let's consider the number of words spoken each day by the average person—words that are spoken purposefully to another individual. Some theorists suggest that men and women speak differing numbers of words daily, whereas others believe the numbers are close. Numerous studies have been done with varying results. Two contradictory outcomes are discussed in an article in *Scientific American*:

About a year ago, Louann Brizendine, founder and director of the University of California, San Francisco's Women's Mood and Hormone Clinic, published *The Female Brain*. One of the most cited gems within its pages was a claim that women are chatterboxes, speaking an aver-

age of 20,000 words per day, nearly three times the mere 7,000 spoken
by men.

A study published today in *Science* reports men and woman [sic]
actually use roughly the same number of words daily.

James Pennebaker, chair of the University of Texas at Austin's psychology department, says he was skeptical of the lopsided stats when he saw
them quoted in an interview with Brizendine in *The New York Times Mag-
azine*. "I read that and I knew it couldn't be true simply because we've
run too many studies," he says, "it just didn't make sense." In fact, he had
been collecting data over the past decade with colleagues at the University of Arizona in Tucson that specifically showed that the sexes are
about equal when it comes to a war of words.

Whether men and women express the same number of words each
day is a discussion for another day. In this chapter I simply want to point
out that whether a person speaks 6,000, 16,000, or 60,000 words daily, a
significant number of words are flowing to, from, and around us. Yet,
how many of those words are taken seriously or remembered? Based on
the number of couples that get divorced, it would seem that the prospect
of words flying thick and fast isn't particularly effective in sustaining
relationships.

It is widely recognized by memory experts that the average person
will forget about half of what is heard within twenty-four hours. Residual
information will gradually dissipate until a person loses most of what has
been heard on a given day within a week's time. When a spouse claims
he "forgot" about a teacher conference for his son despite his wife reminding him a few days before, it's very possible he is right; he may have
forgotten the meeting, just as many people do. Later in this chapter we
will look at ways to enhance memory, but for now the point to be empha-
sized is that more is not necessarily better when it comes to language. In
the case of communication, quality trumps quantity.

VERBAL DENSITY

Many people today communicate with friends and family in brief messages, which may be spoken or written as social media posts or text
messages:

"She went to the store."

"Be home by 11."

"Taking a walk."

Structured as reminders, requests, or commands (using the imperative voice), these statements quickly make their point. Although details may be helpful, they are not always necessary.

For example, does the reader of the note need to know why the writer went to the store or which store? Probably not. Occasionally a reader may become confused when too little information is given, but a follow-up question settles the issue.

However, some spoken or written messages contain overly detailed information, making it difficult for the reader to quickly grasp the meaning. In such cases, "lexical density" should be considered and adjusted for the reader's benefit. Here is an academic definition of this concept by researcher Victoria Johansson:

> Lexical density is the term most often used for describing the proportion of content words (nouns, verbs, adjectives, and often also adverbs) to the total number of words. By investigating this, we receive a notion of *information packaging*; a text with a high proportion of content words contains more information than a text with a high proportion of function words (prepositions, interjections, pronouns, conjunctions and count words).

When planning a message, it is a good idea to include more "content" words than "function words." In fact, you may want to base your message on a solid verbal foundation of a few words, and add only the frills that are truly needed to make the point.

Lengthier messages, detailed in voicemail, e-mail, or letters, sometimes overwhelm readers who simply want to quickly access the message's purpose. Here is an example of a complicated message:

> "Don't forget to take the trash out after work. You know how busy I am, and I simply can't get to it today. If you don't take it out, it will start smelling, and I can't stand the odor."

It is unlikely that most people need that many details to get the point. In fact, it often happens that the main idea can get lost in layers of excessive wording. For important, time-sensitive information, keep the message simple and brief so readers can focus on the main idea.

Requests.

Remember that asking someone to do something requires their time and effort, and possibly the use of their resources. Keep the message brief, clear, and polite, and try to answer questions like what and when, if not why:

A. Ask a relative to take care of a house chore:

"Please sweep the kitchen floor after dinner." (seven words)

Not this:

"Can you sweep the kitchen floor tonight? After dinner would be great. I know you have homework, but it will only take a few minutes." (twenty-five words)

"Can you babysit Friday from 7 p.m. to midnight?" (nine words)

Not this:

"Are you by chance free this Friday, like in the evening? I need a babysitter and was wondering if you can help out." (twenty-three words)

B. Job assistance from a coworker:

"Could you please proofread this report by 5 p.m. today?" (ten words)

Not this:

"I'm not sure this report format is correct. Do you have some extra time to proofread it for me sometime today, maybe before we leave?" (twenty-five words)

"May I leave at 4:30 (instead of 5 p.m.) for a dentist appointment?" (nine words)

Not this:

"I lost a tooth filling and it's really bothering me. I finally got an appointment this afternoon at 5 p.m., which is the latest the dentist will let me come. Is it possible for me to leave early today for the appointment?" (forty-two words)

C. A public favor from an unknown person

"Can a stock associate carry this twenty-five pound bag of soil to my car?" (thirteen words)

Not this:

"I had surgery a month ago and am still not back to normal. I hate to ask, but is there a stock person around that could help? I just need someone to take this heavy bag of soil to my car for me." (forty-three words)

"Do you have change for a twenty-dollar bill?" (eight words)

Not this:

"I usually have lots of smaller bills in my purse, but it looks like all I have is this twenty. Can you by chance cash it for this purchase, or should I use a credit card?" (thirty-six words)

None of the statements are wrong, and these examples could serve as casual conversations. But to get something done quickly, fewer words often facilitate a request. It is surprising how many people feel they must provide an extended rationale, even to those who are uninterested or who do not need additional information. Unless the request is truly out of the ordinary, there is probably no need to elaborate. However, this doesn't mean that accompanying explanations are out of place. Sometimes it is necessary to explain your requests. But on the occasions when you can state a message with less verbiage, why not save your time and the recipient's? Fewer words often create a clearer message.

NECESSARY INFORMATION

Some managers distribute detailed reports or memos that are more confusing than clarifying. Employees struggle to identify the main point(s), which is time consuming and frustrating. Subheadings help to break up a long, complex message. Shorter paragraphs using concrete words will enable readers to quickly grasp the main idea. Readers need to understand what is being conveyed and how they should respond.

I once provided a writing workshop for a steel plant where the supervisor complained that employees did not follow directions outlined in his memos. When I analyzed his writing style and discussed the memos with employees, it became apparent that the supervisor wrote in a rambling style that was hard for employees to follow. Moreover, they were unclear as to what was expected of them in response to the report. With the help of a document template, I assisted the supervisor in organizing his data into categories that made it easier for employees to understand.

Basically, a message comprises three parts: sender, receiver, and message/content. There are many ways to structure a message, but information should be conveyed in ways that readers will quickly grasp. What are we trying to say? What is the best way to present it to recipients? The more efficient our communication style, the better outcomes we can expect.

TWO EARS, ONE MOUTH

When interacting with others, our first impulse is to jump into the word flow. Initially, a greeting exchange includes a sentence or two of no particular significance:

"Hey there."

"How are you?"

"How's it going?"

"What's up?"

The purpose of these expressions is to greet someone and possibly begin a dialogue. If you are not the initiator, it is important to listen and discover the purpose of the conversation, whether face-to-face or by phone. All too often we plunge into a dialogue without adequate preparation. This can lead to misunderstandings or the need to ask questions as the conversation proceeds, wasting time and effort.

Perhaps that is why humans are designed with two ears and one mouth; maybe listening is more important than speaking. When someone starts a conversation, it can be an informal volley of pleasantries at first. Sometimes conversations are great ice breakers or relationship builders. A potential problem is that some people are self-absorbed and when asked about themselves, they release an enormous amount of information, some of which may not be necessary or welcome. Other people are nervous around those they don't know, and they talk nonstop because of anxiety or to fill a conversation gap.

It is a good idea to measure your answers to friendly questions without telling your life story. If your conversation partner mentions a topic, follow up by asking about his or her interest in the topic. You can't go wrong by inviting the other person to share personal thoughts on current events. Many people love to be asked their opinion and will not hesitate to share it.

Being a good listener leads to identifying verbal clues about someone you don't know well. Polite questions about a person's childhood, alma mater, or occupation encourages explanations that reveal his or her personality. Remember not to get carried away in responding to a question or comment. Although it's fine to show enthusiasm, don't be tempted to go on and on about yourself unless the other person specifically asks you to. You don't want to be the one that everyone tries to avoid because of talking too much.

Words have a currency value of their own, similar to money or other assets. Although we may not place a high premium on language and probably spend words more carelessly than a paycheck, we should remember that words have a strong impact on others. They create a permanent impression for years to come—unlike spent funds. Parents, teachers, and employers have unwittingly labeled some for life with thoughtless words. Valuing language as we do other commodities will help us use it wisely rather than squandering words recklessly. Planning should be at least half the effort put into communication, which saves time otherwise spent in clarifying meanings or apologizing for misunderstandings.

WORDS: TOOLS OR WEAPONS?

Many people view communication as a means to an end. In fact, some substitute expressions, gestures, and sounds for words. In a previous chapter we discussed the ways in which silence—partial or complete—can be wielded as a weapon to manipulate others. But words, too, are used to assault recipients, sometimes unknowingly.

Jennifer asks, "Do you want to go see a movie tonight?"

Edward replies with a shrug, "I don't care."

Does he mean he has no preference to go or not go, or is he saying he doesn't have much interest in seeing a movie? If Jennifer doesn't know Edward well, she could interpret his response either way, and the more negative meaning might hurt her feelings. Many hours have been spent pondering a careless statement spoken without much thought.

Some parents nag a child to do (or not do) something. In the cloud cover of numerous words the message gets downplayed, and children learn to tune out something they do not clearly understand. That is why one of the most effective training techniques for toddlers is to use basic one-word commands or short phrases, sometimes accompanied by sign language:

Examples:

Stop.
No.
Don't touch.
Wait for me.

For older children, simple expressions like "I'm sorry" and "I love you" are timeless. Not all messages can be that simple, but when possible, it pays to be uncomplicated. Being nagged about something is not effective. Being asked to do something in clear terms, preferably with a positive or negative consequence in view, can motivate a timely response.

At times I've had to ask for clarification, occasionally more than once, because I could not understand what a person was trying to tell me. There were too many complex ideas to wade through to discern the underlying point. At other times, an explanation was so packed with unnecessary details that it took several moments to sort through them all to get to the heart of the message. I would try to restate what I thought was the main point, only to find I had misunderstood. As the speaker tried again to explain, I remained clueless, leading to added requests for clarification while trying not to antagonize the speaker. When this happens, the wasted time is frustrating to both speaker and listener.

After completing a lay counselor's training program, I met informally with individuals, mostly women, who were seeking guidance about relationship issues. Some could clearly state the problem, whereas others wandered through memories and complaints for several minutes before I could coach them to focus on a specific concern. Granted, some issues require detailed background information, but many do not. Some people are so eager to vent their penned-up emotion that words come pouring out. Although this can benefit the speaker in providing an emotional release, it may delay addressing the issue until a core problem is identified.

Casual conversations among relatives and friends as well as coworkers may need no formal planning. But in messages that are designed to achieve a specific purpose, it helps to plan ahead and decide what the main point will be, as well as any supporting information that might be needed. Everyone's time is valuable, especially in a professional situation, so most people are appreciative when we speak clearly and succinctly.

But there are times when emotions flare and are vented as words—curses, complaints, and criticism. Without thinking, we shovel heaps of damaging words onto someone. In fact, sometimes the emotional floodgates open to unleash massive verbal assaults that not only escalate tensions and lead to conflict, but also overwhelm the listener. The recipient may wonder what led to the deluge and be totally unprepared to respond. Lack of verbal restraint creates chaos rather than communication.

Some of us refrain from speaking up about a troubling situation, only to later burst into a venomous verbal assault when we reach the last straw. Dealing directly with concerns has been discussed in other chapters. The topic overlaps here with the notion that failure to speak up at the right time can erupt in a firestorm of words at the wrong time.

To ensure that the right words are used to convey a clear impression, it pays to plan your discussion by deciding which words to use, and which to avoid, without getting wordy. Budgeting your verbiage and time can increase efficiency. Here are a few tips:

1. Emphasize what should, not what shouldn't, happen. Use modals such as *can, may, ought, will,* and so on, instead of *can't, won't, couldn't* for a proactive approach.

   > Negative examples:
   > We can't work this out if you refuse to change.
   > The problem won't be solved without more money.
   > Positive examples
   > We can work this out if changes are made.
   > The problem can be solved with a bigger budget.

2. Emphasize the action over the person.

   > Negative examples:
   > Your refusal to consider the future is wasting time.
   > You need to start thinking differently.
   > Positive examples
   > Rethinking the future can save time.
   > Thinking proactively could be productive.

3. Outline specific action steps over general goals.
   Rather than simply state a main goal, like "save our marriage," you can accomplish more by developing clearly stated actions that will lead to the goal.
   Examples of action steps for the goal of "save our marriage":

   > a. Spend thirty minutes daily in conversation with each other.
   > b. Overlook a spouse's irritating habit.
   > c. Share one of the spouse's recreational activities— sports, TV, shopping, and so on.
   > d. Overcome a personal habit that irritates the spouse.

4. Listen carefully to others' viewpoints and show respect for differing opinions.
   In preparing a report, a speech, or a presentation, you may want to collect information about and from the proposed audience. For example, understanding the socioeconomic background, education level, and, in some cases, gender ratios of a readership can be useful in tailoring your information. When I make presentations, typically I'll prepare an agenda that is approved by the organization—sometimes enhanced by collecting employees' questions about the topic or goals for the session. Occasionally at the beginning I'll ask the audience what they would like to learn by the end of the session, even if they have already received a prepublished program. When possible, I'll adjust the presentation to encompass their objectives. Otherwise, as has happened to me in the past, I could end up giving a talk that has little direct bearing on the

audience's needs. A questionnaire distributed to registrants ahead of time can collect helpful information for preparing an effective presentation.

> General topic example:
> Male and female communication differences
> Specific topic examples (gleaned from audience's pre-session input)
> Why men and women communicate differently at work
> Why Internet use may vary among men and women
> How clear communication can enhance a marriage

Taking time to find out beforehand what listeners expect can save time to maximize communication success. In some cases, you may have to use more rather than fewer words to clearly state an objective. But the outcome will be worth it and eventually save thousands, if not millions, of words—most of which will be wasted—born out of frustration or misunderstanding. Doing something right the first time saves time.

Language is a valuable human gift that should not be taken lightly. Valuing our vocabularies and conversations is the first step toward using them wisely. If you're tempted to say something, but you're not sure you should, remember the adage, "When in doubt, leave it out."

Corporate leadership has the potential to mismanage communication. Although it is often stated that communication skills are one of the top qualities sought by companies, many leaders have not mastered the art of clear, direct communication, according to Steve Tobak:

> Sure, top executives may give lip service to the idea that they need to communicate and do so effectively, but it's simply not their highest priority. So, things don't come out the way they should, feet end up in mouths, and the next thing you know, it's crisis management time.

We've all seen evidence of corporate miscommunication—specifically, too much communication—in the news. So, if international commerce leaders are beginning to learn the importance of saying less to get more, shouldn't we?

Considering the use of each word and its potential impact on listeners helps us get our ideas across in communication. Notice the way in which you converse with others, or how you respond to someone's question, for an idea of your communication style. If you feel you are too verbose, practice cutting down your sentences by substituting stronger for weaker words.

SUGGESTED STRATEGIES

1. Listen to people around you as they speak. Do you quickly grasp their meaning? If not, how should they rephrase a sentence to make it clearer? Adopt the same approach in your language style if you notice a similar pattern.
2. Review your texts and e-mails. Do they seem rather long and convoluted, or short and precise? If the former, does that seem to be an effective way to communicate with recipients? If not, how could you tighten your style to make it more clear or emphatic?
3. If writing is part of your job, examine some documents you have written. Does the main point come out clearly at the beginning of the document? Will the reader know what the message is going to be about? Are anticipated details or explanations forthcoming in the remainder of the document?
4. Take note if others frequently ask you to repeat or explain something you've said. If they aren't getting it the first time on a regular basis, work on rearranging your sentences to state a main idea at the beginning. Then check to be sure you have clearly explained the idea in the information that follows.

REFERENCES

"Google: There Are 129,864,880 Books in the Entire World." mashable.com, 5 Aug. 2010. Web. 17 Feb. 2014. http://mashable.com/2010/08/05/number-of-books-in-the-world/.

Habash, Gabe. "Average Book Length: Guess How Many Words Are in a Novel." PWxyz *Huff Post Books*, 9 Mar. 2012. Web. 7 Feb. 2014. http://www.huffingtonpost.com/2012/03/09/book-length_n_1334636.html.

Johansson, Victoria. "Lexical Diversity and Lexical Density in Speech and Writing: A Developmental Perspective." *Working Papers* 53: 61–79, 65. Print.

Swaminathan, Nikhil. "Gender Jabber: Do Women Talk More than Men?" *Scientific American* 6 July 2007: n. pag. Web.

Tobak, Steve. "Leaders Should Communicate Less, Not More." FoxBusiness.com, 18 Feb. 2014. Web. 27 Feb. 2014. http://www.foxbusiness.com/industries/2014/02/18/leaders-should-communicate-less-not-more/?intcmp=fbfeatures.

TEN

Words on the Web

Electronic communication has been around for decades and continues to reach into the lives of billions of people daily. Cell phones, texting, e-mail, and faxes are widely used for personal and professional interactions by busy moms and businesswomen. Face-to-face conversations of the past are now conducted via video conferencing and face time. But how effective is electronic communication?

Although traditional in-person communication is still valuable because of the added ability to interpret body language (meta-communication) and gestures as well as expressions, there are numerous advantages to electronic communication, including flexible scheduling, preview time, editing options, and sharing capabilities. However, the downside to mechanical chat includes the uncertainty of conveying or interpreting emotions and losing momentum in a conversational exchange because of disruptions of time and place. Web-based communication and cell phone use help to promote clear-cut understanding, but there are potential drawbacks. Direct and honest communication can be subverted—inten-

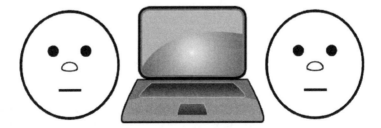

Figure 10.1.   Digital distancing

tionally or otherwise—thus, electronic communication should be used carefully.

Busy women who multitask as wives, moms, employees, caregivers, and volunteers make numerous contacts in a typical day. Cell phones, text messages, e-mail, instant messaging, blogs, bulletin boards, social media, and video conferencing are just some of the channels through which communication flows, in addition to the traditional desktop phone or home landline.

Electronic devices are effective for communicating in social and peer relationships but may diminish family interactions. Clutching a cell phone 24/7 and texting during family time is just plain rude. In any social gathering it is increasingly common to find people engaged in two, three, or more conversations simultaneously:

- Face-to-face
- Cell phone
- Texting
- Tweeting
- Social networking

As we come of age and venture into the world—increasingly through computer and cell phone portals—we experiment with a variety of media. The tantalizing option of instant connection may render users somewhat unable to fully evaluate the pros and cons of digital communication. Certainly, a quick text or Facebook post saying "I'll be home later" is easier than trying to locate a spouse or child and offer a personal explanation. But a brief written message, no matter the medium, can raise more questions than it answers. Too few words or too little context may easily contribute to miscommunication. Have you ever received a text message from an unknown source? You may have spent considerable time digging through previous text records to locate the number and identify the sender. Occasionally someone accidentally sends a message to the wrong recipient, causing confusion and, in some cases, alarm. As with all forms of written communication, it is important to double-check transmission data for accuracy.

Electronic media, whether on cell phones or the Internet, should not be used hastily or carelessly. A message should be sent only through a medium clearly understood by the user and receiver.

MOBILE (CELL) PHONES

A *Time* article indicated that "of the world's estimated 7 billion people, 6 billion have access to mobile phones." *Internet World Stats.com* states that in second quarter 2012 there were 2,405,518,376 Internet users in the world. A growing sense of connectedness is helping to address isolationism and promote global interaction, but at what cost to personal relationships?

A mobile phone is a status symbol, not just a communication device. Lacking one subjects many women to jokes about being out of date. Because so many people use them, those without cell phones may experience a sense of social ostracism and be unable to keep up with the communication flow. Some cell phone users are obtaining increasingly sophisticated features and applications. Communication has never been so exciting, nor has it caused so many headaches for those who are trying to keep up with the Joneses and maintain a hip image.

Cell phones can be used for numerous functions. An employee on her lunch break can sit with coworkers in a restaurant while using her phone to conduct any combination of activities, deftly moving from one to the other, maintaining conversational flow with several people at once.

Unless one is expert in multitasking, however, those conversations are apt to be brief, superficial, error-riddled, and repetitive. Women often enjoy the challenge of juggling several conversations simultaneously, in addition to paying bills and updating their social network status. But how meaningful is this continual stream of cell phone usage? Because much can be lost in translation in conversations among varied users, care should be taken to correctly interpret digital messages to prevent misunderstandings. Potential problems often arise from slang, which can be used in any communication format. For example, let's say someone texts a friend with the offer to babysit her toddler so the friend can go shopping. If the friend texts back, "That's okay," does it mean the offer is welcome—or unnecessary? A face-to-face conversation would fill in the blanks by allowing the sender to observe the recipient's facial expression or body language. Similarly, the use of emoticons can be confusing to those who are less familiar with them.

Heavy cell phone use may interfere with other endeavors. For example, in academic arenas, a recent study at Kent State University (Ohio) revealed that students with high levels of cell phone use tended to have lower GPAs and higher anxiety levels:

> Their analysis showed that cell phone use was negatively linked to GPA—the higher the cell phone use, the poorer the grades—and positively linked to anxiety—higher cell phone use was linked to higher anxiety. (Paddock)

Although a number of factors may be involved in the study's conclusions, it is possible that students who are intensively engaged with cell phones during class time or homework activities are not wholly involved with course content. Half-hearted attention to discussion can prevent even the best students from successfully meeting learning outcomes. In applying this pattern to a busy mother of a preschooler, if she is frequently using her cell phone, is she being the most effective parent possible?

Child safety may become an issue for moms who continually use their phones while simultaneously monitoring young children's activities, such as taking a bath or playing outside.

An article by Helen Lee Lin in *Scientific American* details a study that suggests merely having a cell phone nearby—without using it—may hinder the development of meaningful relationships:

> Przybylski and Weinstein asked pairs of strangers to discuss a moderately intimate topic (an interesting event that had occurred to them within the last month) for 10 minutes. The strangers left their own belongings in a waiting area and proceeded to a private booth. Within the booth, they found two chairs facing each other and, a few feet away, out of their direct line of vision, there was a desk that held a book and one other item. Unbeknownst to the pair, the key difference in their interactions would be the second item on the desk. Some pairs engaged in their discussion with a nondescript cell phone nearby, whereas other pairs conversed while a pocket notebook lay nearby. After they finished the discussion, each of the strangers completed questionnaires about the relationship quality (connectedness) and feelings of closeness they had experienced. The pairs who chatted in the presence of the cell phone reported lower relationship quality and less closeness.

Awareness of and access to a cell phone may serve as a visual reminder of a virtual world at our fingertips, thus diverting attention from limited in-person conversations. A smartphone can be used to transact most if not all of our typical daily activities. Having a phone handy contributes to a sense of security, or it may have the opposite effect—creating insecurity unless one is habitually using its many features. I've noticed at countless meetings one or more persons using a cell phone to conduct various activities, like balancing a checkbook, shopping online, or networking with friends on social media. Occasionally, but not often, I'll notice a cell phone, untouched, sitting on a desk in front of a person.

The prolific use of cell phones is profoundly impacting the ways in which we communicate. Gone are the days when a landline was "busy" or "out of service." Although either can happen with cell phones, these events are less common. When they do occur, a voicemail message can be left if desired, unless texting is available, which then becomes an alternate communication medium. Increased access to other people via technological devices is likely affecting our style of interaction because we don't have to make an appointment or schedule a meeting for an important discussion or meeting:

> The cell phone also reshapes the social norms of talking in public places. It has enormous impact on existing social institutions. With the expansion of the Internet on cell phone devices, the nature of social contact has transformed into creating new "technosocial situations" where people are always available. (Nurullah 23)

Instead of thoughtfully planning a conversation while waiting to dial a number or answer the old table-top desk phone, it is easy to get caught up in a rapid-fire exchange of information—or, more likely, emotions—using a handheld cell phone without clearly planning the conversation. When someone is always "available," it is tempting to contact that person day or night with a message that may be unclear or incomplete, which can waste time and lead to annoyance. Think of midnight texts, e-mails, or social networking posts you have received. Isn't it often the case that people think differently at midnight than at midday? Our inhibitions drop, emotions may flare, and logic is sometimes clouded by fatigue. Then, when a message has been carelessly sent, it is impossible to call it back, revise it, or cancel it.

In professional communication, fast-paced dialogue sometimes leads to errors stemming from missing details or contacting the wrong person—particularly when using speed dial or smartphones. Instant access can be tremendously helpful, but it can also lead to problems that eventually cost time and money. For example, a department's new trainee who has the supervisor's office number on speed dial can quickly call with a question and receive prompt feedback. Of course, without the phone number the new employee can simply go to the supervisor's office for help, but that may be blocked by the supervisor being away from the office or busy with other employees. Given a choice, most people will use a phone before getting up to physically seek information. The downside to this situation is that an uncertain employee may get in the habit of calling a nearby coworker because it is convenient or may ask a question before being fully ready to discuss the issue, requiring time-consuming follow-up interactions.

Although much of this depends on human nature and personal idiosyncrasies, it can be generally agreed that the speed and convenience of cell phones, including texting, may unwittingly encourage ill-timed or premature interactions that subsequently require additional explanations or clarifications.

Moreover, because electronic communication is available 24/7—that is, we can e-mail, text, or tweet a message at 2 a.m. for someone to read the next day or whenever desired—it is tempting to compose messages when tired, distracted, or ill. Although face-to-face conversations are limited to both parties' scheduling availability, and landline phones that ring audibly usually occur at convenient times, texts and e-mails can be sent anytime and accessed by the receiver when desired. This ready availability of communication may hinder the thoughtful preparation of a meaningful message and instead foster careless exchanges that are later regretted.

SOCIAL NETWORKING

Facebook, Instagram, LinkedIn, Pinterest, and other social and business networking sites are proliferating. Increased numbers of users are flocking to these sites to find old friends, make new friends, and stay in touch with current friends.

According to "Worldwide Social Network Users: 2013 Forecast and Comparative Estimates," nearly one in four people worldwide used social networks in 2013. The number of social network users around the world rose from 1.47 billion in 2012 to 1.73 billion this year, an 18 percent increase. By 2017, the global social network audience will total 2.55 billion.

A *TechCrunch* article indicates that 73 percent of U.S. adults use social media networks (Lunden). With the rapid pace of social media evolution, it seems unlikely that most users share uniform understanding and usage of these networks. If that is true, then it is highly likely that misunderstandings occur between those with uneven levels of knowledge and experience, especially between generations or cultures. For example, a college student who stays in touch with hometown friends and family may post to her social networking site several times a day and check the posts of people she knows who are likewise online, whereas her father seldom checks his social networking account. Thus, their connection will be tenuous unless they use other communication media as well.

A social networking service is a wonderful way to connect with people that you might not otherwise talk to, such as distant relatives or former friends. Catching up online is convenient and cheap. But if exchanges are random or few, shared information may be limited and generalized. Those that stay in touch frequently are more likely to exchange meaningful details of their lives.

But a social network account can also tempt members who don't know each other well to project a fake persona for egotistical purposes such as flirting in a pretend romance (especially by shy or married users), deceiving underage victims, or swindling unaware victims. Some job hunters also misrepresent themselves online by fabricating their credentials or references.

However, communicating with someone via a social networking site offers distinctive advantages for building honest and open relationships. Posting photos, vital statistics, and "statuses" can reveal a great deal about a person, including information that may change from day to day. Spiritual beliefs, occupation, and hobbies are some of the usual facts that can be found on personal Web pages at sites such as Facebook, for example. Professional networking sites provide opportunities to list job history, achievements, awards, and career goals, among other things. Members should keep in mind that once posted, their personal information in many ways belongs to the Website, and they may later have difficulty permanently retrieving everything that has been shared. It is essential to read the Website rules and policies before becoming a member and posting personal information.

Because many people live several "lives" simultaneously—wife, mother, employee—it is important to realize that public information may be accessed by anyone, except that which is intentionally kept private. So if an employee of a company is moonlighting as an independent consultant, posting that information on her site may allow the primary employer to view it and raise questions about the ethics of holding two positions, as some companies hold strict policies in this regard. Similarly, there are numerous cases of people whose activities in one aspect of their lives—for example, as exotic dancer—may impact another aspect—such as a teaching job. Although some believe diverse activities should not interfere with each other, the fact remains that disparate parts of our lives can and do intersect, often with unexpected consequences. This leads to the question of how direct one should be in posting personal information online. Each of us must answer that question individually and thoughtfully.

Even when members do not initially post highly personal details of their lives, getting involved with other members may naturally lead to online exchanges where personal information is shared. One cannot be too careful in screening those who ask questions that require revealing answers. Information posted online may be impossible to recall; thus, it is best to offer only the facts that you don't mind anyone seeing—ever. Web-based words have a way of floating in cyberspace forever. They can show up unexpectedly during a search of someone's name or relevant keyword. Never post anything that you may later regret.

Honest, direct, and forthright communication can be used in social networking in getting to know a person "virtually" before meeting in person. Exchanging factual information typically found on a resume with someone who appears to be trustworthy can facilitate a meaningful introduction between two people. Moving from an objective position to a more intimate level of interaction is often the next logical step. However, it is easy to deceive someone by inventing an identity for unethical use, referred to in popular culture as "catfishing." An unscrupulous member who poses as something he or she is not to scam others is, sadly, not uncommon. That is why you should take time to validate a new person's identity through shared acquaintances or through information that can be checked. For example, if someone claims to be an usher at the community playhouse on Thursday nights, you could probably call or visit the theater to find out for sure.

Social networking sites, creating a parallel virtual world, construct an environment that is conducive to illusions and masquerades. Unseen entities compose untrue identities to scam unsuspecting victims. All of this potentially leads away from direct communication into the realm of surreal interaction that is similar to visiting a funhouse. As you walk through its mazes and peer in the mirrors, you get a distorted sense of reality that can be amusing or scary. At least you know a funhouse is not real, whereas on the Web, it can be difficult to know what is real and what is not.

Electronic communication has become the norm. A careless approach to Internet or cell phone interactions will lead to haphazard results. We must use these media efficiently and safely for optimal results.

SUGGESTED STRATEGIES

1. In professional situations, use template responses for consistency. You don't want to create an automatic response that sounds artificial, but you can readily customize responses by topic or title. Examples:
   a. Responding to requests for information
   b. Acknowledging receipt of submissions or applications
   c. Rejections for various reasons
2. When using voicemail and video messaging, remember to speak clearly and plan your message before delivery. This will help to avoid rambling thoughts and forgotten details while keeping the message on track, saving time and preventing confusion.
3. Electronic communication usually is stored in ways that can be later retrieved. Never send a written or spoken message that you are not comfortable making potentially public at some future point. Possible risks include a security breach or the forwarding of a message to unknown persons.
4. Plan and preview your message before sending it. This is one of the distinctive advantages of electronic communication over face-to-face interaction.
5. Use mobile phones appropriately and politely. Don't overlap with simultaneous communications, and do not use when engaged in other activities or conversations.
6. Review text messages before sending them. Use emoticons sparingly.
7. Be cautious when using social networking sites. Never divulge personal information to someone you don't know. Become acquainted before agreeing to meet in person, and meet in a public place, giving family members the details.
8. Remember that anything posted on the Internet may be around forever. No matter how hard you try to remove a message or photo, it can be difficult if not impossible to completely retrieve.

REFERENCES

"Internet Users in the World." Internet World Stats.com, 30 June 2012. Web. 11 Mar. 2014. http://www.internetworldstats.com/stats.htm.

Lin, Helen Lee. "How Your Cell Phone Hurts Your Relationships." *Scientific American* 4 Sept. 2012: n. pag. Web.

Lunden, Ingrid. "73% of U.S. Adults Use Social Networks, Pinterest Passes Twitter in Popularity, Facebook Stays on Top." *TechCrunch* 30 Dec. 2013: n. pag. Web.

Nurullah, Abu Sadat. "The Cell Phone as an Agent of Social Change." *Rocky Mountain Communication Review* 6: 19–25, 23. *Academia.edu*. Web. 21 Mar. 2014.

Paddock, Catharine. "Cell Phone Use Linked to Lower Grades, Anxiety." *Medical News Today* 9 Dec. 2013: n. pag. Web.

"Social Networking Reaches Nearly One in Four Around the World." eMarketer.com, 18 June 2013. Web. 11 Mar. 2014. http://www.emarketer.com/Article/Social-Net-working-Reaches-Nearly-One-Four-Around-World/1009976#y8HHcSp8y1AvsXLw.99.

Wang, Yue. "More People Have Cell Phones Than Toilets, U.N. Study Shows." *Time* 25 Mar. 2013: n. pag. Web.

Conclusion

Make It Count

A few months ago my friend Rita invited me over to watch a video, one we both wanted to see.

"Sure," I said. "What time?"

"Oh, I'm flexible. Just let me know what works for you," she said.

We agreed that sometime between seven and nine would suit us both, and I would touch base with her later.

Close to seven, I called Rita to ask if she was ready to see the movie.

"Oh, I just finished watching it," she replied, "since I had nothing else to do. But we can rent another video."

Deflated, I suggested we postpone our movie night. I had been pumped up to see that particular film, and Rita's watching it without me was disappointing. Had I somehow missed a communication point that seeing it together was optional rather than planned?

I don't think I misunderstood. Rather, Rita takes a flexible approach to communication and planning, whereas I tend to be more precise. In learning to accept differences in communication style, I understand the importance of detailed interactions to avoid misunderstandings.

What I've learned about being "direct" is that there are "degrees" of directness. Some people are more straightforward than others. Just when you think you've been as clear as possible, someone will misunderstand, and you start questioning the communication process and how the breakdown occurred.

We live in an imperfect world. Wires get crossed. By learning to speak up and speak out, we can better understand each other by removing the guesswork. Then we will enjoy greater success in personal and professional interactions. However hard we try, being direct isn't always easy for everyone. But it can get easier with effort.

INDIRECT OR UNDECIDED?

You probably know people who are hesitant to make decisions. They show interest in an activity but resist making a firm commitment. This can range from something as simple as dinner plans to choosing a marriage partner. Although occasional indecision is understandable and often commendable, chronic indecision makes it tough on those who need clear answers. Indecision can come from uncertainty, fear, or many options, as well as other reasons. But it is important to communicate clearly even about hesitation. Asking for clarity can help to reduce misunderstandings. For example, if your supervisor asks you to update a file, you may want to ask about the priority order of that task if other work has already been assigned.

Timeliness is another critical factor in decision making. "Can I get back to you on that by tomorrow morning?" is an example of postponing a decision in a clear way. This response sets a firm deadline while allowing time to consider the issue. A vague reply like "Let me give it some thought" leaves the hearer hanging without a specific timeline for getting an answer. Sometimes an open response is necessary when dates or details are unknown. But when possible, definitively state an expected response or date.

It's natural to have ambivalent feelings about whether to watch a movie, go shopping, or take a nap. But it's impolite to keep others waiting. Release them from the courtesy of awaiting your reply by saying something like, "Thanks for the invitation. I'm not sure if I feel up to it this afternoon. Let's try for another day." An aunt and uncle in my friend Erika's family are habitually undecided about accepting holiday dinner invitations. Aunt Paula says, "We'll let you know soon" but fails to RSVP until the last minute. Then, after accepting an invitation, Aunt Paula and Uncle Norm frequently change plans at the last minute or arrive late. Keeping their options open is more important to them than considering potential inconvenience to the hostess. In this situation, it would be helpful for Erika to politely request a firm commitment by a certain date because she is not happy with the uncertainty of her relatives' participation.

One way that job supervisors can be indirect is when they delay in responding to employee questions. For example, a college dean who fails to promptly address faculty requests for authorization may cause them to miss grant deadlines, conference registrations, or research opportunities. A factory supervisor with a delayed response to employee questions may slow the production process. An elementary schoolteacher who neglects to acknowledge her young pupil's waving hand may have to deal with a toileting accident or a failed math concept.

Although a vague promise to "respond as soon as possible" may be legitimately the result of a supervisor's hectic schedule, it is discourteous to keep others waiting indefinitely for important information. Instead, a frantic supervisor may need to reevaluate her schedule to ensure that duties are handled competently with respect for all. Even if an important decision must be delayed, a quick note to acknowledge an employee's question is courteous and professional.

Vagueness is another kind of indirect communication. With promises to find answers to employee questions or consult others who need to be involved, a supervisor who does not follow up within a reasonable time can complicate a situation. If delays are inevitable, an estimated time frame should be provided. In fact, the supervisor should periodically check back on prior questions to get a status update and ensure the situation is being responsibly handled.

Related to vagueness is estimation. Although estimating cost and time is a normal part of a project forecast, extended estimates are problematic. Some people toss out estimates without much thought, leading to confusion and mishaps.

"I can tutor your child in math for a few weeks, and it won't cost much at all," Alicia, a young mom of a toddler offers her neighbor. Then, after working with the girl for a month, three nights a week, totaling twenty-five hours, she asks her neighbor for $250, charging $10 an hour. The tutoring rate is fair, but the unsuspecting neighbor may be taken by surprise, not expecting to pay a hefty sum over the course of a few weeks. Alicia did not mean to be deceptive or take advantage of her neighbor. A careless offer with nonspecific information led to unexpected results. When possible, it is a good idea to provide specific details as to what to expect and thus prevent unpleasant surprises.

An unwillingness to say no is another way in which some people communicate indirectly. Fearing to hurt someone's feelings, a kind-hearted supervisor might string an employee along without a firm "no" in response to a request. For example, a motivated employee asks for a meeting to discuss a raise and possible job advancement. The equally motivated and budget-minded supervisor avoids the "showdown" she believes will result from the meeting.

"We'll talk about it soon," the supervisor says, without any real intention of meeting. It is better to say, "Sorry, there's no money in the budget right now for raises," than to keep a worker waiting and then exasperate her when the meeting and raise do not materialize.

The same is true for parenting children. Moms who know they are going to say "no" should not tell their kids "we'll see" or "maybe" in response to a request. If a delay is necessary to decide, parents should make this clear: "I'll discuss it with Dad tonight and let you know tomorrow." This response sets a good example for children to follow rather than foster mistrust in parents' noncommittal responses.

Occasionally, an indirect approach may be useful, for example, when you don't want to overstep boundaries or be perceived as overbearing.

Those situations should be carefully evaluated to ensure that an indirect manner is indeed the best approach. An employee who suggests an annual morale-boosting event may want to phrase it delicately if the boss is known not to appreciate suggestions or if the budget is tight. However, in regular circumstances this type of statement can probably be stated directly without being intrusive.

Similarly, a woman who continually voices her views or makes decisions for the parents' group she belongs to might be better appreciated if she restrains her opinion to let everyone have a say. Hearing everyone's ideas is generally more productive than letting one dominant person lead.

TOO DIRECT

Is it possible to be too direct?

That can happen. Some people say exactly what they think, whenever they feel like it. However, without considering the context, the target audience, and the purpose of the message, language that is excessively direct often borders on being offensive.

Years ago, I belonged to a study group that included a fortyish single woman, Joanie, who was known for her blunt, outspoken manner. Joanie was intelligent, but also, as it seemed to me and others, somewhat socially insecure. That combination of traits may have been the basis for her extremely direct manner. Joanie would ask pointed questions, such as someone's age, even when she knew that person did not wish to speak of it publicly. Sometimes she would confront a member of the group about something that person said or did. Although not exactly antagonistic, Joanie was nevertheless not the most comfortable gal to be around, and as a result, she did not enjoy widespread popularity. But a core group of five or six of us who got to know her rather well eventually relaxed our guard and began to appreciate her personality strengths while overlooking what we perceived to be as Joanie's conversational weaknesses, especially being overly direct.

Even further along that end of the spectrum are those who seem to lack the social graces altogether. They are often blunt and to the point, typically overstepping social conventions to have their say. In fact, their manner can be more abrupt than that of someone like Joanie. This person will walk up to you, say something excessively direct—often without context—and leave you wondering how to respond. Questions like "Where do you work?" and "How many times have you been married?" make many people uncomfortable. Fortunately, a casual comment can ease the tension: "I'm in the hospitality business" or "How did you know I was married?" can help to offset the initial discomfort. This level of abruptness may be the result of an emotional, social, or physical condition and probably is not intended to be rude.

Certain kinds of leaders develop an autocratic style of communicating that is often one-sided and marginally demeaning. They sometimes speak in loud, strident voices or a mocking tone, or use staccato phrasing that utilizes action verbs:

"Sweep this floor *now*," an irate factory supervisor yells to a nearby worker.

"I want the report by five p.m. today—not when you decide to show up tomorrow morning," the manager insists while passing a busy employee's desk.

You don't have to guess what these people are thinking; they tell you in no uncertain terms. However, their brusque manner can be offensive and sometimes puzzling, leaving the listener to wonder if she was joking. All too soon, employees will learn that this dictatorial style is meant to be taken seriously, and it frequently leads to dislike if not conflict. Those with a direct communication style at work can soften the blow with a brief smile or low-key tone.

In personal relationships, being direct all the time may take a toll on a couple's emotions. There are times when being indirect is desirable and perhaps necessary, as when consoling someone for a loss or trying to make amends. An indirect approach is often helpful with sensitive people, or when discussing topics that may be fraught with tension, such as money, religion, or politics. It is usually a good idea to avoid topics that lead to conflict, unless there is a compelling reason to pursue the discussion.

Being indirect may mean not getting involved in delicate conversations, or not offering an opinion unless it is asked for. There are times when it is wise to merely state reasons without emphasizing an opinion, letting the evidence speak for itself and allowing listeners to draw their own conclusions. For example, when a husband asks if his work pants still fit him, you could tell him they're too tight, if you want to be direct. Or if you prefer a more indirect approach, tell him they fit snugly and let him apply his own interpretation. Often, directness versus indirectness comes down to a matter of words.

SPEAK UP

At a time when women need to speak up to defend their rights and responsibilities, learning to speak directly is a valuable asset that should not be overlooked. Beginning with everyday situations, we can learn from and teach other women how to speak up for what is truly important, from personal freedoms to political action. Learning how to use important communication tools can make the difference between success and failure. Although there are certainly times to use indirect speech or no words at all, the bottom line for any communication is clarity. Thus, effective interaction interprets the dynamic roles of speaker, listener, and message to work toward the projected goal of meaning. Advancing to global self-expression is the next step, as evidenced in the courageous life of Pakistan teenager Malala Yousafzai:

> Pakistan's renowned teenage activist Malala Yousafzai spoke with VOA Deewa about International Women's Day. She was asked what advice she had for women and girls around the world. The teen activist called on women to speak up.
>
> "My message to women and girls all around the world is that they should speak up for their rights. Because when you do not speak up our voices are not heard, but if we want to see a bright future then we must speak."
>
> In 2009, Malala Yousafzai challenged the Taliban in her native Pakistan and their ban on girls attending school.
>
> In 2012 she was attacked by gunmen as she made her way home aboard a school bus. Yousafzai remained in a coma for 10 days, eventually completing her recovery in the United Kingdom. Today, the 16-year-old continues to fight for equality in educational opportunities worldwide.

In 2014, the International Women's Day theme is "Equality for women is progress for all." Issues involving gender equality, women's empowerment, and human rights are among the core objectives. Women must first learn to speak up clearly—and directly—about personal concerns and objectives in their natural domains—home and work. When they do, they will be empowered to take a stand on far-reaching goals that impact us all.

In conversations that matter, we should all take a few minutes to think about what we want to say. Then we must consider who we will be talking to and his or her specific needs. Finally, it is important to decide how to deliver the message effectively to elicit the response we hope to receive. Arranging words and sentences is like playing Scrabble by using the creative process to render the most meaning. With effort and ingenuity, you can learn to say what needs to be said in a way that will render desired results.

REFERENCES

"Teen Activist Malala Urges Women to 'Speak Up.'" *Voice of America*, 8 Mar. 2014. Web. 17 Apr. 2014. http://www.voanews.com/content/teen-activist-malala-urges-women-to-speak-up/1867041.html.

Bibliography

Andersen, Erika. "How Great Leaders Deliver Bad News." *Forbes* 6 Mar. 2013: n. pag. Web.

Ashkenas, Ron. "First Rule of Management: No Whining." *Forbes* 7 Nov. 2012: n. pag. Web.

Bernstein, Elizabeth. "For a Nation of Whiners, Therapists Try Tough Love." *Wall Street Journal* 15 May 2012: n. pag. Web.

Bies, Robert J. "The Delivery of Bad News in Organizations." *Journal of Management*: n. pag. *Journal of Management*. Web. 19 Jan. 2014.

Bloom, Linda, and Charlie Bloom. "The Cost and Benefits of Emotional Honesty." *Psychology Today* 12 Dec. 2011: n. pag. Web.

Bouris, Karen. ""How Vulnerability Holds the Key to Emotional Intimacy." *Spirituality and Health* 1 Nov. 2012: n. pag. Web.

Bowers, Michael J., and Margaret McCarthy. "'Language Gene' More Active in Young Girls Than Boys." *Science* 22 Dec. 2013: n. pag. Web.

Cacioppo, John T., James H. Fowler, and Nicholas A. Christakis. "Alone in the Crowd: The Structure and Spread of Loneliness in a Large Social Network." *Journal of Personality and Social Psychology* 1 Jan. 2009: 977-991. 984. Web.

Carter, Sherry Bourg. "High Octane Women." *Psychology Today* 27 Apr. 2011: n. pag. Web.

"Charm." *Merriam-Webster.com Dictionary*, n.d. Web. 15 Jan. 2014. http://www.merriam-webster.com/dictionary/charm.

Cornblatt, Johannah. "Lonely Planet." *Newsweek* 20 Aug. 2009: n. pag. Web.

Dawson, James R. "Communicating through Silence." ADI Marketing, 9 Aug. 2012. Web. 20 July 2013. http://amarketing.com/2012/08/09/communicating-through-silence/.

Draper, Michael, Rachel Pittard, and Michael Sterling. "Self-Disclosure and Closeness."

Eco, Umberto. *A Theory of Semiotics*. Bloomington: Indiana UP, 1979. Print.

"Genesis 3." *The Bible*. Bible Gateway. Print.

Goldberg, Eleanor . "Yemeni Girl Who Evaded Child Marriage, Says She'd 'Rather Die' Than Get Married Off." *Huffington Post* 22 July 2013: Video.

Goleman, Daniel. "Emotional Intelligence." N.p., n.d. Web. 16 Dec. 2013. http://www.danielgoleman.info/topics/emotional-intelligence.

"Google: There Are 129,864,880 Books in the Entire World." mashable.com, 5 Aug. 2010. Web. 17 Feb. 2014. http://mashable.com/2010/08/05/number-of-books-in-the-world/.

Gregore, Carolyn. "Why You Should Care about Having Friends at Work." *Huffington Post* 9 July 2013: n. pag. Print.

Habash, Gabe. "Average Book Length: Guess How Many Words Are in a Novel." PWxyz *Huff Post Books*, 9 Mar. 2012. Web. 7 Feb. 2014. http://www.huffingtonpost.com/2012/03/09/book-length_n_1334636.html.

Halken, Beth. "Whining: Why It Happens and What To Do About It." babycenter.com, 1 Mar. 2012. Web. 15 Jan. 2014. http://www.babycenter.com/0_whining-why-it-happens-and-what-to-do-about-it_63630.bc.

Hanover College, 18 Apr. 2008. Web. 7 Oct. 2013. http://vault.hanover.edu/~altermattw/social/assets/w08papers/Draper_Pittard_Sterling.pdf.

Hodge, Robert , and Gunther Kress. *Social Semiotics*. Ithaca: Cornell UP, 1988. Print.

"How Can I Find Someone To Just Listen To My Problem and Maybe Advise Me What To Do?" *Ask.com*, 11 Mar. 2011. Web. 23 Oct. 2013. http://www.ask.com/answers/6435081/how-can-i-find-someone-to-just-listen-to-my-problem-and-maybe-advise-me-what-to-do.

"Humoral Theory." Contagion: Historical Views of Diseases and Epidemics, Harvard University, n.d. Web. 16 Dec. 2013. http://ocp.hul.harvard.edu/contagion/humoraltheory.html.

Ibsen, Henrik. *A Doll's House*. Project Gutenberg, n.d. Web. 15 Jan. 2014. http://www.gutenberg.org/catalog/world/readfile?fk_files=3275005&pageno=1.

"Internet Users in the World." Internet World Stats.com, 30 June 2012. Web. 11 Mar. 2014. http://www.internetworldstats.com/stats.htm.

Johansson, Victoria. "Lexical Diversity and Lexical Density in Speech and Writing: A Developmental Perspective." *Working Papers* 53: 61-79, 65. Print.

Jones, Patricia. "The Silent Treatment: A Form of Abuse." Dove Christian Counseling, n.d. Web. 31 July 2013. http://www.dovechristiancounseling.com/SilentTreatment.html.

Krauss, Robert M.. "The Psychology of Verbal Communication." N. Smelser, and P. Baltes, eds. *The International Encyclopedia of the Social and Behavioral Sciences*. Columbia University. 1 Jan. 2002. Web. 8 Feb. 2014. http://www.columbia.edu/~rmk7/PDF/IESBS.pdf.

Lin, Helen Lee. "How Your Cell Phone Hurts Your Relationships." *Scientific American* 4 Sept. 2012: n. pag. Web.

Llopis, Glenn. "Getting Past 4 Common Workplace Fears." *Forbes* 24 June 2013: n. pag. Web.

Lunden, Ingrid. "73% of U.S. Adults Use Social Networks, Pinterest Passes Twitter in Popularity, Facebook Stays on Top." *TechCrunch* 30 Dec. 2013: n. pag. Web.

Maloni, J.A., and R.M. Kutil. "Antepartum Support Group for Women Hospitalized on Bed Rest." *AM J Matern Child Nurs* 25: 204-10. NCBI. Web. 9 July 2013.

Markway, Barbara and Greg Markway. "Shyness is Nice." *Psychology Today* 28 Aug. 2011: n. pag. Web.

Matsumoto, David, and Hyi Sung Hwang. "Reading Facial Expressions of Emotion." American Psychological Association, 1 May 2011. Web. 11 Feb. 2014. http://www.apa.org/science/about/psa/2011/05/facial-expressions.aspx.

McCrae, Fiona. "Women Talk Three Times as Much as Men, Says Study." *Daily Mail* 28 Nov. 2006: n. pag. Print.

Mielach, David. "Silent Women: Why Women Don't Speak Up." *Business News Daily* 20 Sept. 2012: n. pag. Print.

Mohindra, Vinita, and Samina Azhar. "Gender Communication: A Comparative Analysis of Communicational Approaches of Men and Women in Workplaces." *Journal of Humanities and Social Science* 2: 18-27. *iosr journals*. Web. 19 Dec. 2013.

Neubert, Amy Patterson. "Cold Shoulder, Silent Treatment, Do More Harm Than Good." Purdue University News, 27 July 2005. Web. 15 July 2013. https://news.uns.purdue.edu/html3month/2005/050727.Williams.exclusion.html.

Nurullah, Abu Sadat. "The Cell Phone as an Agent of Social Change." *Rocky Mountain Communication Review* 6: 19-25, 23. *Academia.edu*. Web. 21 Mar. 2014.

Paddock, Catharine. "Cell Phone Use Linked to Lower Grades, Anxiety." *Medical News Today* 9 Dec. 2013: n. pag. Web.

Palmer, A. "Self-Disclosure a Leading Factor in Not Seeking Therapy." American Psychological Association, 1 Sept. 2003. Web. 7 Oct. 2013. http://www.apa.org/monitor/sep03/factor.aspx.

Parpart, Jane. "Choosing Silence: Rethinking Voice, Agency, and Women's Empowerment." Gender, Development, and Globalization Program. Center for Gender in Global Context, 1 July 2010. Web. 20 July 2013. http://gencen.isp.msu.edu/documents/Working_Papers/WP297.pdf.

Payne, Karen. "Caltech Counseling Center." Caltech Counseling Center, n.d. Web. 25 Oct. 2013. http://counseling.caltech.edu/general/InfoandResources/Shyness.

"Professional Women: Vital Statistics." Fact Sheet 2010: Department for Professional Employees, n.d. Web. 24 Oct. 2013. http://www.pay-equity.org/PDFs/ProfWomen.pdf.

"Psychologists." Occupational Outlook Handbook, United States Department of Labor, n.d. Web. 16 Dec. 2013. http://www.bls.gov/ooh/Life-Physical-and-Social-Science/Psychologists.htm.

Ralston, Jeannie. "Lies In Marriage: What We Don't Tell Our Husbands." *Parenting* 1 Jan. 2012: n. pag. Web.

Riggio, Ronald E. "Women's Intuition: Myth or Reality?" *Psychology Today* 14 July 2011: n. pag. Web.

Rinpoche, Dzogchen Ponlop. "Relationships: Riding Your Emotional Rollercoaster." *Huffington Post* 7 July 2010, sec. Lifestyle: n. pag. Print.

Segal, Jeanne, Melinda Smith, and Lawrence Robinson. "Emotion Communicates! The Powerful Role Emotions Play in All Relationships." UMHS EAP, n.d. Web. 13 Dec. 2013. http://www.sitemaker.umich.edu/um-aaop/files/emotion_communicates.pdf.

Sholar, Monica Hersh Khetarpal. "Jurors' Perceptions of Gender-Biased Linguistic Differences." *William & Mary Journal of Women and the Law* 10: 90-136. Web. 13 Dec. 2013.

Smith, S. E. "Psychiatrisation: A Great Way To Silence Troublesome Women." this ain't livin', 13 Aug. 2010. Web. 22 Apr. 2013. http://meloukhia.net/2010/08/psychiatrisation_a_great_way_to_silence_troublesome_women/.

Smyth, Joshua M., Arthur A. Stone, Adam Hurewitz, and Alan Kaell. "Effects of Writing about Stressful Experiences on Symptom Reduction in Patients With Asthma or Rheumatoid Arthritis: A Randomized Trial." *JAMA* 281: 1304-1309. *JAMA Network.* Web. 2 July 2013.

"Social Networking Reaches Nearly One in Four Around the World." eMarketer.com, 18 June 2013. Web. 11 Mar. 2014. http://www.emarketer.com/Article/Social-Networking-Reaches-Nearly-One-Four-Around-World/1009976#y8HHcSp8y1AvsXLw.99.

Swaminathan, Nikhil. "Gender Jabber: Do Women Talk More than Men?." *Scientific American* 6 July 2007: n. pag. Web. .

"Teen Activist Malala Urges Women to 'Speak Up.'" *Voice of America*, 8 Mar. 2014. Web. 17 Apr. 2014. http://www.voanews.com/content/teen-activist-malala-urges-women-to-speak-up/1867041.html.

"The 5 Love Languages Explained." Personality Cafe, 21 Aug. 2012. Web. 11 Feb. 2014. http://personalitycafe.com/articles/112444-five-love-languages-explained.html.

Tobak, Steve. "Leaders Should Communicate Less, Not More." FoxBusiness.com, 18 Feb. 2014. Web. 27 Feb. 2014. http://www.foxbusiness.com/industries/2014/02/18/leaders-should-communicate-less-not-more/?intcmp=fbfeatures.

Wang, Yue. "More People Have Cell Phones Than Toilets, U.N. Study Shows." *Time* 25 Mar. 2013: n. pag. Web.

"Whine." Merriam-Webster Dictionary, n.d. Web. 15 Jan. 2014. http://www.merriam-webster.com/dictionary/whine.

"Why Adults Whine and How to Stop Them." *The Buffalo News* 1 Dec. 2012, sec. City and Region: n. pag. Print.

Why Women Don't Speak Up at Work. Perf. Jennifer Hartstein, Ivanka Trump. MSN youtube, 2013. Film.

Zadro, Lisa. "Silent Treatment: Uncovering the Nature and Consequences of Ostracism." *Association for Psychological Science Observer* 26: 768-774. *Association for Psychological Science Observer.* Web. 1 July 2013.

Index

About the Author

Debra Johanyak is professor of English at the University of Akron Wayne College. She is a frequent writer and speaker on how women talk to people in their lives. She has published three previous books.